Everything <u>Else</u> You Need to Know When You're Expecting

Everything <u>Else</u> You Need to Know When You're Expecting

The New Etiquette for the New Mom

Paula Spencer

ST. MARTIN'S GRIFFIN ⚞ NEW YORK

Design by Maureen Troy

ISBN 0-312-24337-5

First Edition: March 2000

10 9 8 7 6 5 4 3 2 1

For George, who is simply the best

Contents

Timing. Ways to tell. Handling gun-jumpers. Siblings. Details.
Plus: Creative Ways to Tell; Do's and Don'ts for Dads-to-Be

When you're not yet pregnant. Nosy questions. Old wives' tales.
Unwanted advice. Gory details. Labor stories. Belly-rubbing.
Plus: Really Awful Questions; Don't Believe Them!; But These Old Wives' Tales Are True!; Do's and Don'ts for Grandparents-to-Be

When to start. Basics. Borrowing clothes. Shopping. Dressing for work. Formal dressing. Casual dressing. Post-baby.
Plus: When the Invitation Says . . .

Rest rooms. Nausea. Doctor's appointments. Switching health professionals. Finding out the baby's sex. In transit. Smokers.

Complaints. Social obligations. Bed rest. Miscarriage. Aprés-
baby helpers. Water breaking. Guardians.
Plus: Great Escapes; Do's and Don'ts for Best Friends

Telling others. Maternity leave. Small talk. Absences. Eating.
Work showers. How long to work. Labor at work. The big news.
*Plus: When They Say . . . You Can Say . . . ; Do's and Don'ts
for Colleagues*

Hosting a shower. Guests. When to hold. Invitations. Location.
How many? Who has a shower? Work showers. Grandmother
showers. Themes. Gifts. Twin gifts. Games. Menu. Imperfect
gifts. Return gifts? Thank-yous.
*Plus: Clever Corsages; Baby-Shower Table Favors; Shower
Refreshments*

Conventions. Junior. Middle names. Surnames. Telling others.
When partners disagree. Namesakes. Nicknames. Unusual
names. First dibs. Criticism. Indecision.
*Plus: Sources of Inspiration; More Naming Traditions; Take the
Name Test; Ten Things One Never Should Say About a Baby's
Name*

Attendees. Birth party. Labor support. Out of control. Filming
birth. Thank-yous. Spreading the word. Celebrations. Circumcision. Hospital stays. Problems at birth.
Plus: More Ways to Celebrate Birth; Circumcision: Yes or No?

The basics. Timing. Types of announcements. Examples. Un-
usual announcements. Newspaper.
*Plus: On-Line Birth Announcements; Ways to Word It; More
Ways to Tell the World*

Acknowledgments

I certainly would not be minding my manners if I didn't properly thank all of the people who helped me write this book. And so, a bouquet of grateful thanks to each of the following individuals:

First, my sincere appreciation to the many experts (including, of course, many mothers) who shared their own questions, answers, customs, ideas, and time: Patti Anderson, Mary Hopkins Bailey, Dawn M. Barclay, Chris Cardone, Jennifer Evans, Jody Kozlow Gardner, Dorothy Foltz-Gray, Melanie Haiken, Anne Krueger, Beth Levine, Leslie Dunn Levine, Jeanne Martinet, Kathleen McCleary, Mary Niepokuj, Karol Patyk, Laura Patyk, Maura Rhodes, Ellen Robinette, Anne Goodwin Sides, Beth Schwartz (senior rabbi at Temple Beth-El, Knoxville, TN), Cherie Serota, Karin Sparks, Kathy Spencer, Cherie Spino, Susan Salmon Trotman, Catherine Wald, Donna Young Whitley (pastoral coordinator of Sacred Heart Church in Norfolk, VA), Jody Wright, and Nancy Young, as well as the many others with whom I've had chance conversations. I'd also like to recognize the manners mavens whom I've interviewed on various occasions in the past and whose legendary knowledge informs this book, especially Marjabelle Stewart Young, Letitia Baldridge, and Judith Martin.

My special thanks to the publishing pros who shared and

shaped the book's vision. They are my agent, Loretta Weingel-Fidel, and my editor at St. Martin's Press, Jennifer Weis.

On a much more personal level, credit must go to the people who "brought me up right," my parents, Eleanore and Sylvester Patyk.

Finally, my chief prodder, editor, advisor, and steadfast champion has been my husband, George. Without him, there would be no book. Nor, of course, would there be a Henry, Eleanor, Margaret, and Page—our four special children whose pregnancies, births, and infancies inspired this book.

Introduction

"It's got hiccups! Feel!" Without thinking twice, I grabbed my co-worker's hand and placed it on my big, hard, eight-months-pregnant belly. He blanched. Then he fled the room mumbling something about a phone call he had to make right away.

Now, I like to think of myself as a polite person. But clearly, putting my (childless, male, uptight) colleague in an awkward position wasn't one of my most considerate moves. **During my four pregnancies, I continually found myself in similarly strange new situations,** uncertain what was the "right" thing to do. Would it be so terrible if I cut in a mile-long rest-room line during intermission at the theater? What's the protocol for borrowing maternity clothes? Must I let strangers pat my belly? What *would* I do if my water broke right then and there on my hostess's new rug?

The need for a book like this struck me while I was on temporary bed rest when pregnant with my third child. Lying there, helplessly, I wondered if, when friends inquired how they could help, I could direct them to the skyscraper baskets of laundry. (Yes, I learned, if I asked nicely.) Around the same time, my husband and I were wrangling over the question of whether a second-born son could be his namesake, if we'd passed over that idea for the firstborn. (Yes again, I discovered; why not?)

At first glance, the idea of a guide to maternity manners may sound a tiny bit totalitarian. Shouldn't a woman great with child be allowed to do as she darn well pleases? Doesn't she have enough to worry about, between her expanding front, her shrinking bladder, and the varicose veins snaking up her legs?

As a mother of four who writes about pregnancy and parenthood for a living, I'll be the first to insist that mothers-to-be deserve a wide latitude (no pun intended) about most matters. **Nevertheless, there's a graceful way and a klutzy way to do nearly everything—and that includes having a baby.**

Besides, pregnancy and new parenthood are rife with strange new experiences to figure out—the sorts of things you mull over with friends, rather than your doctor. Most pregnancy books ignore them; most etiquette books barely skim the surface. When do you tell the boss you're expecting a baby during the busy season? What's the difference between "junior" and "the second"? Between a guardian and a godparent? How do you word a birth announcement (and does e-mail count)? Are you supposed to courteously serve tea to visitors who come to see the newborn when you're still bleary-eyed and can feel every single episiotomy stitch?

Nor are expectant mothers the only ones with the questions. Partners wrangle over baby names. Friends want to give showers. Relatives visit. Mothers-in-law dole out advice. And all of the above search for just the right gift.

Think of this not as a rule book, but as an idea book.

It's crammed with answers to all those nagging little questions that crop up during that blissful, bizarre, upside-down year of pregnancy and new parenthood. The solutions are not always black-or-white. Rather, they're informed suggestions, based on the foundations of proper etiquette, generations of custom, modern reality, common sense, and the wonderful wisdom of dozens of other mothers who have gone through it all before you.

Happy pregnancy, happy baby, and good luck with all those thank-you notes.

Everything <u>Else</u> You Need to Know When You're Expecting

1

Spreading the News

Congratulations, you're pregnant! Along with all the new physical and emotional changes you're about to undergo, you're also on your way to the strange new world of maternity manners. The questions start, literally, as soon as your doctor (or, more probably, your little home-test stick) provides the confirmation: To tell, or not to tell? Whom to tell? When to tell? Letting the world know you're expecting a baby is delicious fun. Here's how to get things off to a good start.

TIMING

What's the proper time to announce a pregnancy?
No one blinks anymore when couples spread the word the minute the home test turns positive. (Or even sooner, as when they reveal that they're "trying.") Being pregnant is incredibly exciting, after all. But there are good reasons to hold off a few weeks, as people did before the advent of the instant, superaccurate home pregnancy test.

First of all, the risk of miscarriage is highest during the first twelve weeks of pregnancy (the first trimester, or twelve weeks counting from the first day of your last menstrual period). In the terrible, but unfortunately not uncommon, event of a miscarriage, all of the people who have been told about the pregnancy will wonder, a few months down the road, what's happened. Unless the couple goes back and informs everyone about their misfortune—not a fun task—the friends are placed in the awkward position of worrying but not wanting to ask directly. Then, when they learn of the unhappy news, they will feel bad too.

Yes, we live in a sped-up, instant-gratification, zap-mail, drive-through-dry-cleaners kind of world. We want it all, right now. But birth is a mystery with a pace all its own. You have nine months ahead of you. Savor the news. Keep it to yourself for a little while. Many couples find that sharing this special secret draws them especially close.

You are rightfully ecstatic about the baby growing within you, but the rest of the world will be far more interested in the actual baby. Tell too early, and you spend the next eight-and-a-half months hearing, "Haven't you had that baby *yet?*" If you think nine months of pregnancy is an eternity, imagine how it stretches for interested observers, who don't have first-hand experience of your aches and pains and kicks to keep things fascinating. Couples who spread the news the day they find out shouldn't be disappointed if their friends and relatives seem a bit bored by the subject as the weeks wear on.

Especially at work, the later you wait, the better, so your physical state won't distract others from your performance. (See Chapter 5, "Pregnant at Work.") Unless you make it so, an impending birth is really nobody's business until you start to show.

Women who can't stand to keep such a momentous secret might want to let a close friend, a sister, or their mother in on the news, ideally someone who's already a mother herself. This gives the mom-to-be an outlet for her excitement and complaints, as well as a source of advice, without having to tell the world.

Is it better to wait to tell other people until after a doctor confirms the pregnancy?

If you're gung ho to spread the word immediately, there's little point in waiting for an official medical confirmation. Performed properly, home pregnancy tests are now considered 99 percent accurate. A doctor cannot foretell whether you're likely to miscarry or not. Note: if however, an early ultrasound (around six weeks into the pregnancy) detects a heartbeat, your odds go up tremendously that you will remain pregnant.

WAYS TO TELL

Is there a preferred way to say it?

Choose the words you're comfortable with: "Guess what? Bob and I are expecting a baby next June!" This phrasing is discreet, inclusive of your mate, and also preempts the inevitable next question, "When?" Most people aren't squeamish any more about the word "pregnant," thank goodness, so you can also just blurt out "I'm pregnant!"

Single women and lesbian couples who are expecting will inevitably raise lots of eyebrows. Bold friends may go so far as to ask, "How?" or "Who's the father?" Needless to say you are under no obligation to disclose any details. This is no time to be coy. Simply say, "I'm sorry but that's private." Or, "I'd rather not go into that." And change the subject.

Can I send printed announcements that we're expecting?

Printed, no. Written, yes—though only in the most casual way, that is, to mention your pregnancy in a letter to a friend. Ideally, this is the sort of news most people like to hear about in person or by phone, so they can give you a congratulatory hug or at least get an immediate reply to the question of "When?" Save printed announcements until the egg is hatched—which is a far greater accomplishment than merely fertilizing it.

What about sending retail cards that mention where we're registered for baby items, as a way to spread the news?
Let me make this very clear: You may not send these pre-printed cards to inform friends and relatives that you are expecting. What's more, you may not even send them when you are nine months along and due any day. You may not even give them to a friend to slip into the baby-shower invitations.

Cards provided by retailers to herald your news and the fact that you are part of their gift registry—no matter how cute they are—are naked expressions of greed. To the recipients of such notices, they are a demand for a gift. But gifts can never be demanded, only gratefully received and acknowledged. No one who receives such a notice is under any obligation to do anything with it. Besides, if you've just found out you're pregnant, it's far too early to think about baby's gifts, unless you're the eager grandma-to-be who's been itching to go baby shopping for the past ten or fifteen years.

Is there a certain preferred order in which to tell people?
The very first person to be informed is the father—even if he's out of town, unreachable by phone, or on the outs with you. And that's true even if you can't get hold of him and are itching to tell your best friend or your mom. (I once FedEx'd my husband the little test stick with the bright blue line on it. No other message.) Of course, if your mate is standing right next to you watching the test results, you can move on down the list.

Beyond the daddy-to-be, let the depth of your relationships be your guide. It's nice if Mom and Dad are fairly high up on the list. You don't want them to hear the news from a distant relative, even if your relationship hasn't been especially close lately. After all, this is their grandchild.

How should I break the news to a friend who's struggling with infertility?

Nobody likes to cause misery. But a true friend will be happy for you, whatever her personal situation. It's tempting to bend over backward to avoid offending her by *not* telling her at all. But don't put it off so long that she hears the news through the grapevine or guesses it herself. *That's* uncaring.

Do show sensitivity to a friend's fertility problems by telling her in a one-on-one meeting, rather than in front of a large gathering. Acknowledge that you're nervous about telling her in the light of her difficulties. She'll eventually share your joy, though perhaps not immediately. (Of course, spare her such details as that you conceived on the first try.) Don't be surprised, however, if she cries or seems cool to you for a while. Don't take it personally—she's not reacting to your situation so much as her own. Even if she's thrilled for you, she may need a little time to absorb the news.

Creative Ways to Tell

Want to let the daddy-to-be or your parents know about your pregnancy in a special way? Whether the following ideas are corny or heartwarming depends a lot on your personality. Either way, they're exuberant. Some ideas:

- Serve a baby-sized dinner: Baby carrots or miniature corn, baby lima beans, new potatoes, baby-back ribs, and popcorn shrimp. Top it off with pickles and ice cream.
- Wrap up a bib that says, "I love Daddy" or "Grandma's Little Angel."
- Wait for the next holiday (major or minor) to spring the news, and say, "I've got a wonderful present for you for Groundhog Day . . ." If it's Father's Day or Grandparent's Day, all the better!
- Give a baby-themed picture frame or Brag Book, with a note: "Picture to follow around (your due date)." Or place a sonogram image in the frame.
- Tell your husband in the same place where he proposed.
- Buy a high chair into which you place a baby doll and a note: "Feed me. Love me. I'm yours!"
- Buy some baby clothes, put them in a bag, and ask, "Would you like to see my new outfits?"
- Look in stores that sell baby gifts for items or cards with fitting slogans about babies. (When I found out about my fourth child on Christmas Day, I gave my husband a tin cup on which had been printed: "Babies are such a nice way to start people.")
- Form the letters B-A-B-Y with bread dough and bake; ask your mate to check the bun in the oven.
- Go out to dinner. Prearrange for dessert to be served with a pacifier garnish.
- Hang an extra stocking on the mantel (if it's Christmas)
- Pop in a CD or cassette tape of lullabies in the car for your partner's morning commute.
- Send flowers with a message.

- Wrap up a baby doll, preferably one that cries.
- Send a videotape of the ultrasound.

HANDLING GUN-JUMPERS

How do I respond to people who ask if I'm pregnant, before I want to tell?
Let's set aside the intrusiveness of their question for a moment. If you say no, and you are, then you're lying, which is not usually very comfortable for most of us. But that doesn't mean you should be badgered into confessing something so personal before you're ready.

When I was pregnant with my first child, I was determined to wait the full twelve weeks of my first trimester before breaking the news. I thought I was doing a great job of it, too, until one afternoon when the woman in the next office blurted the question. "Why do you ask?" I stammered, trying to keep my hand from floating up to my belly.

"Well, you're wearing your skirt untucked, and I've noticed you stopped drinking coffee," she replied in a triumphant, "ah-ha!" tone. (Office busybodies don't just hear everything, they're incredibly sharp-eyed, too.) Determined that this woman would not hear my happy news before my own mother did, I just laughed something like, "Well, I read that untucked shirts are very big this winter. And as for caffeine, don't you think we all drink too much of it for our own good?" My colleague probably saw through both sidesteps, but she also got the message that she had intruded too far.

You could also turn the tables, and say, "Why do you ask? Do I look fat?" This deflects the embarrassment off of you and onto your questioner. If she has the nerve to persist and say, "Well, a little," it's tempting to retort, "Well, I was thinking the same about you." But that wouldn't be very nice. So instead toss off a wry. "Thanks for the compliment," or, "Well, I'd better go take a walk, then"— and do.

SIBLINGS

When's the best time to tell older siblings? We want them to be in on the secret but don't want them to blab to everyone else.
When to tell a child that a baby brother or sister is about to join the family depends on the child's age. Some pointers:

- *Toddlers*: A toddler has no sense of time. He or she may even be oblivious to your growing belly (until your lap completely disappears, anyway). You can talk about the baby growing in your tummy but don't expect the news to register completely. Be low-key. It's usually best not to emphasize the forthcoming baby until your last weeks of pregnancy. (And don't even bother bringing up the finer points of biology. When I was nine months pregnant with my second child, my twenty-one-month-old son poked me and asked, hopefully, "You got a ball in there for me?") Even with preparation, a toddler is apt to be amazed when you actually bring a baby home.

    Minimize feelings of displacement by moving the older child out of his crib or into a new bedroom at least four to six weeks before you're due, or wait until a couple of months after the birth.
- *Preschoolers*: Kids ages three to five are a bit more aware

of what's going on around them than young toddlers are. They're apt to notice your swelling belly and increasing fatigue. But times moves painfully slowly for them, especially when special events and "gifts" (like a baby brother or sister) are involved. It's therefore best not to tell a preschooler until you begin to show, or better still until he or she notices. Read books about babies and how they are born, let your child practice with his or her own baby doll, and consider enrolling in sibling-preparation classes, offered at many hospitals. Let your child feel the baby move. Let him or her help you pick out a special toy or nursery items for the new born. Curb expectations, toward the end, by reminding your child that the new baby will be small and helpless, not a ready-made playmate.

- *Older children*: Whenever you choose to break the news, certainly school-age children deserve to know about a pregnancy before outsiders do. The best strategy is to tell your child just before you're ready for others to hear. Most school-age kids ask detailed questions about how babies grow and are born; answer them honestly, in simple terms. Look for age-appropriate books. Let them help you make things ready for the baby.

DETAILS

Should I announce the fetus's gender and name or keep them secret?

It's your call. Now that prenatal tests such as ultrasound and amniocentesis have made it possible to find out your baby's gender before birth, the majority of expectant parents these days want to have this information. So, in turn, do their friends and family. And so the first question many moms-to-be are asked, after "When are you due?" is "What are you having?"

It's certainly your prerogative to buck this trend and enjoy the grand mystery of birth as it was originally intended. But even if you choose to know—maybe because you want the baby to seem as real as possible or because you're the type who just likes to have all the facts—you may want to think twice before sharing that info with the world. Take shower presents, for example. If you announce that you're having a girl, you're apt to receive countless frilly baby dresses, all size three months. Few women let loose in a baby department knowing that they are buying for a baby girl will be able to resist these tiny pretties. And should you announce the baby's name while he or she is still in utero, brace yourself for a volley of criticisms or alternative takes.

Some people actually act irritated when told that you don't plan to learn the gender. When one woman's family members complained they wouldn't know what to buy for her baby, she replied, "Just assume it's human and work from there."

Of course, people will be excited by word of the baby's arrival regardless of how much they know about him or her in advance. But it does add an extra dollop of excitement when they can say to one another, "It's a boy!" rather than, "Oh, Arthur Alexander finally arrived . . ."

Do's and Don'ts for Dads-to-Be

DO cuddle next to her with your hand on her belly as often and for as long as she wants you to.

DO NOT *recoil when you see the baby somersault under*

her navel. It's not a scene out of Alien *and no, it won't burst out and devour your fingertips.*

DO ask "How are you feeling today?"
DO NOT *ask, "Why are you crying?" She doesn't know either.*

DO notice—and comment on—how pregnancy hormones have made her hair thick and lustrous.
DO NOT *notice—and comment on—the way those same pregnancy hormones have made her skin erupt like an adolescent's.*

DO gush over the layette's tiny ribbon-trimmed underthings the way you once gushed over her tiny black-lace-trimmed underthings.
DO NOT *ask what they cost or roll your eyes and say, "Heck, you could have just cut some armholes and neck holes in a pillowcase. The baby won't know the difference."*

DO listen empathetically to her complaints about backaches, bloating, and all-through-the-night trips to the bathroom, no matter how often she repeats them.
DO NOT *complain yourself—especially about how all the focus on her and the baby makes you feel like a third wheel. You are.*

DO let her hog the extra pillows to cushion her body at night.
DO NOT *count (out loud, anyway) how many weeks it's been since the two of you had sex.*

DO realize that morning sickness lasts morning, noon, and night.

DO NOT *grill Italian sausage, boil cabbage, or douse Mongolian Fire Oil on a wok full of Szechwan pork and scallions in her presence.*

DO mail her funny postcards of babies that say on the back, "See you soon!" **DO NOT** *forget to send—at bare minimum—a card for Mother's Day, should it fall during her pregnancy.*

DO praise her pulchritudinous voluptuousness. **DO NOT** *use descriptions of her like "tank," "Greyhound Scenicruiser," or "Goodyear blimp."*

DO go shopping with her for a new maternity dress in her last trimester, when she moans she's sick of her wardrobe. **DO NOT** *tell her you've seen better-looking sacks in a grocery store.*

DO remain calm on the drive to the hospital so that you can help her through her breathing exercises. **DO NOT** *stop at Burger King on the way for fortifications and tell the order-taker, "My wife's having a Whopper!"*

DO hold her hand during labor, mop her forehead, and prepare to possibly be ignored or insulted. **DO NOT** *turn on the television in the labor room. Even if your team is in the finals.*

DO dial your in-laws' number from the hospital after the baby's born to tell them the news before you call your own parents. **DO NOT** *forget that new moms need as much TLC as pregnant ones. Maybe more.*

DO smile agreeably when she suggests having another baby because the first one's so adorable.

DO NOT *do anything more than smile agreeably—at least not until you've changed the first thousand diapers.*

2

Busybodies

One of the least anticipated aspects of pregnancy for many women is the effect that your new state has on others. Veteran mothers begin doling out advice by the paragraph. Your husband monitors your every move. Your friends tell stories that make pregnancy sound more like a horror flick than a blessed event. And if that's not dismaying enough, wait until you start to show! You're asked questions more personal than anything Oprah would dare, even during sweeps week. Perfect strangers reach out to grope your midriff in ways that would ordinarily get them arrested.

What's a nice mom-to-be supposed to do, especially when she's had (and heard) enough? Read on.

WHEN YOU'RE NOT YET PREGNANT

I'm not pregnant yet, but what do I say when I'm asked: "Are you trying?"
Some blunt people go around asking straightforward questions all the time. Others assume (incorrectly) that questions surrounding procreation are fair game for couples of a certain age and relationship status. For many people, such inquires have become benign, cocktail-party fodder, something to ask besides "What do you do?" and "Are you married?" Even ordinarily discreet folks tend to lose all pretense of civility when

it comes to babies. Though the questioners may be probing out of love or good intentions, they are nevertheless way out of line. Very personal questions are impolite, and never more so than when they surround one's sex life.

You're not obligated to answer any questions you don't want to, just to be nice.

Say, "Excuse me?" to signal that your questioner has overstepped his bounds. Another appropriate response: "I'm sorry but that's a difficult and personal question. I'm sure you'll understand if I don't answer it." But if he persists, lightly take evasive action: "Well even if we were, it's certainly not something I want to go around talking about."

NOSY QUESTIONS

What do I say if I'm asked, "Was it an accident?"
It will surprise many people, who have come to regard all matters concerning babies as a matter of public interest, that to ask details about a baby's conception is unspeakably rude. It's rude because it is intrusive and prying, and concerns a subject that's just about as private as you can get. On top of being nobody's business, it cruelly implies that if the answer is yes, the baby must not be as cherished or wanted as a baby who was planned.

If you're feeling charitable, you might arch your brows at your questioner, and say, "You know Freud said there is no such thing as an accident." Or you could say, "Why? Does it matter?" (Watch the backpedaling that then takes place.) But you're well within your rights to simply deliver the iciest stare you can muster, and say, incredulously, "I beg your pardon?"

It's only slightly more tactful for someone to ask, "Was it planned?" But the net implications are the same.

Unfortunately, such questions have become so common-place that they've become part of the vernacular of preg-nancy. Although one might be tempted just to chalk them up to another tiresome toll of being pregnant, none deserves answers unless you really care to provide them. It's the ques-tioner who's out of line, not you.

It's never necessary to answer a personal question, no mat-ter whether the questioner is your mother, your social supe-rior (like an elderly aunt) or a professional superior (your boss). You don't even have to answer your best friend. *Ex-ception:* It's always a good idea to answer your health-care practitioner as thoroughly as possible. Unlike your mother and your elderly aunt, he or she is not just prying. There are underlying medical reasons behind a doctor's or nurse's ques-tions.

Below are some other questions commonly heard in pregnancy, and ways to handle them.

. . . "When are you due?"

Most women would not consider this a nosy question. And most are more than happy to give a direct answer. This can be vague ("at the end of summer") or precise ("My due date is September 7"). Asking, "When are you due?" is a benign way to show interest in a pregnancy. The questioner may also have a practical motive for the question, for example, to get a sense of when the woman will stop attending a club meeting or participating in her car pool.

Because the inquiry is personal, however, it's therefore bet-ter asked by acquaintances than strangers. One woman, tired of being asked over and over by people she didn't know, finally snapped, "I'm so sorry to disappoint you. I'm just really fat." By the time you're in your last trimester, you're entitled to a little levity.

... "Do you want a boy or a girl?"

Your questioner is asking you to publicly choose sides, setting yourself up for later guilt if you give birth to a child of the sex that you weren't hoping for. Even if you and your partner have a preference, it's not anyone else's business. Best to lean on that old chestnut: "We don't really care, so long as it's healthy."

... "Did you take fertility drugs?"

Personal questions are always impolite, but in this particular case, don't automatically assume nosiness. "Respond by saying, 'Why do you ask?' " suggests Maureen Doolan Boyle, executive director of Mothers of Supertwins in Brentwood, New York, herself the mother of triplets. "The person could be asking because they're struggling with infertility, and you could then offer helpful information and resources."

If they're obviously just a busybody, saying, "Why do you ask?" ought to clue them that they've strayed into inappropriateness. Never answer a question you don't wish to.

... "Is it a boy or a girl?"

This question assumes (or knows) that you've already had a prenatal test—ultrasound, chorionic villus sampling (CVS), or amniocentesis—that has divulged the fetus's sex. The query has grown in popularity because these tests have become so common. Still, it's an intrusive thing to ask. If you do know and want to tell, go ahead. (Be prepared. Next they'll ask, "What names have you picked out?" or "Will you have him circumcised?") Otherwise, the best answer is "We don't know." Even if you do.

... "Are you worried about birth defects?"

This question is as ignorant as it is nosy. Every mother worries, on some level, about whether she'll deliver a perfect baby. That doesn't mean she wants to go around talking about it. Older expectant mothers, especially, tend to hear this question because the statistical risk of some kinds of birth defects rises after ages thirty-five or forty. That doesn't excuse it, either. Best response: "There are a million things for pregnant women to worry about. But I find it more helpful to focus on positive thoughts."

. . . "Is pregnancy hard on you?" or "Aren't you too old for this?"

Whether phrased in a veiled or a blatant way, these zingers are aimed at a mom-to-be's age. (Younger women who are prematurely gray hear them, too.) Considering how commonplace first-time motherhood has become for women in their thirties and forties it's slightly surprising that such questions should even come up. But they do. Women in midlife pregnancies will also hear their share of jokes ("Maybe the baby will be born with gray hair") and gentle digs ("I'll have all my kids out of the house by the time your baby is just starting nursery school!").

Respond with the truth: "I feel great, thanks." Or, "If I wasn't too old to get pregnant, I don't think I'm too old to *be* pregnant." You could also point out some of the many recent examples of older first-time moms. For example, TV actress Adrienne Barbeau delivered her twins by natural childbirth at fifty-one, and Jane Seymour was forty-four when her twins were born. Kim Basinger became a mom at forty-one. Newswoman Connie Chung adopted her son when she was forty-nine. Examples of famous moms having subsequent children in their forties are even more abundant: Caroline of Monaco at forty-two, Christie Brinkley at forty-four, and Susan Sarandon at forty-five, to name a few.

Humor can help brush off such questions, too. One forty-two-year-old, whose three other children were already in high school, liked to quip, "We were just checking to see if everything was still working."

... "Aren't you worried about how much your life will change?"
Older expectant parents and groundbreakers who are first in their crowd to procreate tend to be the recipients of this one. Perhaps the question is well meant. When your lifestyle is conspicuously child-free—dinners out, spontaneous travel, softball leagues, and the like—well-wishers may genuinely be trying to picture your future *en famille*. Or they may just be envious. Either way, you need only reveal as much information as feels comfortable.

Easy out: "Well I'm sure our life will be different, but life is all about change, isn't it?"

... "Who's the father?"
Social disdain for single mothers has all but disappeared in the last twenty-five years or so. Even lesbian partners having a baby has stepped off the tabloid talk shows into everyday life. But curiosity about the particulars remains a hot topic. Everyone's bound to speculate—although that doesn't give them permission to do so to your face.

Whether your baby's arrival was planned or unplanned, how many details you wish to share with others is up to you. And that most certainly includes how you happened to become pregnant in the absence of an obvious answer. Use discretion in deciding which details you'll make public, however, and to whom. Realize that not everyone may share your moral outlook. Also resist using an innocent baby to proselytize about your own lifestyle choices.

Possible responses:

- *Evasive:* "Thanks for your interest. You'll be sure to get a birth announcement when the big day gets here."
- *Firm:* "That's a private matter."
- *Humorous:* "That's between the baby and me." (Or, "That's between the baby and us." Or, "I can't remember. He was in the band.")

... "Why are you drinking coffee/eating a donut/crossing your legs?"

Ah, the pregnancy police. A swollen belly attracts more watchdogs than a prison. They're all around you, ready to growl when you make a move that they consider the least bit unhealthful, teeth bared (in a helpful smile) to nip bad habits in the bud. These unsolicited exhortations are usually directed to a pregnant woman's diet or exercise habits, although everything's a potential target, including her posture and her state of mind.

Such interferences are usually as well intentioned as they are annoying. That does not excuse them, however. Nagging is never nice. Not even when it's meant to instruct someone in the error of her ways. Not even when the welfare of a new human being is at stake. If you're participating in an activity that the other party firmly believes to be wrong (drinking coffee, eating a donut, crossing your legs) it is wrong of them to point this "error" out to you. Informing someone of her shortcomings is not only presumptuous and supercilious—it's also often misguided. Maybe the coffee is decaffeinated—anyway, the occasional cup is not thought to be harmful. Squishy glazed donuts lack nutrients, but there's no law against consuming them in pregnancy. And never mind the discussing the position of someone's legs. Right or wrong, it's definitely none of anyone else's business.

Often raids by the pregnancy police are based on misconceptions, outdated information, or a lack of knowledge about the individual mom-to-be's health. For example, someone who has never jogged before would not be advised to do so during pregnancy, but a healthy marathoner can probably continue a modified schedule of runs approved by her physician.

Some of these incessant interrogators are just plain mean, spoiling your day in a selfish attempt to show off their own pregnancy know-how (whether they know anything or not). Worst of all, these ever-so-helpful souls actually expect you to be grateful for the unsolicited assistance.

You know your own self and your doctor's orders better than anyone else does. Don't let intrusive nags turn your pregnancy into public property. Offer a cool "Thanks for taking an interest in my pregnancy, but I assure you everything's just fine." And continue on with the donut or the coffee. Or fall back on, "My doctor says it's okay." Refuse to be intimidated.

It's especially awkward when your own partner joins the cop squad. If he's willing to forgo drinking wine because you can't, that's wonderful. If he volunteers to cook you tasty protein-packed meals with green leafy vegetables on the side, that's charming. But when he starts grabbing chocolate-chip cookies out of your hand and making you step outside the room whenever he runs the microwave, it's fair to say enough is enough. It may be his baby, but it's your pregnancy, and your body.

If you are engaging in a behavior that is generally agreed by the medical community to be unwise during pregnancy— drinking, doing illegal drugs, and smoking come foremost to mind—technically it would still be off base for an observer to point this out to you. Surely you already know the dangers of such behavior, and nagging is unlikely to change it. Realize, however, that those who intervene over such serious matters are doing so because they love you—and your unborn baby. So let me issue a preemptory nag: If you're engaging in behavior that *your doctor* has advised against, please please stop during your pregnancy. Nine months isn't that long.

Really Awful Questions

Some questions are the absolute Mount Olympus of nosiness. The all-purpose answer to prying is to say, "I *beg* your pardon?" with all the astonishment you can muster. But just in case your questioner misses the point and repeats the question, try these replies:

When They Say . . .　　　　### You Can Say . . .

When They Say . . .	You Can Say . . .
"So are you throwing up all the time?"	"Not all the time—not at the moment, for example."
"How much weight have you gained?"	"Since when?"
"Don't you think the world is overpopulated already?"	"The more the merrier."
"Haven't you learned about birth control yet?"	"I only discuss birth control with my partner, thank you."

What They Say . . .	*You Can Say . . .*
"Can you still see your feet?"	"Why? Are they doing something I should be aware of?"
"Is sex better now?"	"Why do you want to know?"
"Why on earth are you having another one?"	"Thank you for your interest in our growing family."
"Do you realize that you'll be fifty when your child is in fourth grade?"	"Yes, and when he's seventeen, I'll be sixty, and he can turn me on to all the new tunes."

OLD WIVES' TALES

Can I correct someone who tells me an old wives' tale that's clearly wrong?
Folk wisdom is maddening when you know better. Be pregnant long enough (who isn't?) and you'll hear the one about how eating strawberries will cause red birthmarks or swimming in water over your navel is sure to drown your baby. Swallow the urge to sputter, "That's crazy," which is neither courteous nor constructive.

Instead, consider the source, and her motives. Your mother, grandmother, and all the other old wives who spout such tips mean well. It's their way of showing they care. Their clucking and sharing allows them to participate vicariously in your pregnancy. Thank the helper for her interest, or say, "Really? I hadn't heard that," and let it go. Distract the advice-giver, while still encouraging her involvement, by soliciting her input about something more benign, such as her opinions about baby names or nursery decor.

Above all, be nice. No one appreciates hearing that his or her knowledge is thirty years behind the times, even if it is.

How can I politely ignore advice that seems dangerous?
Maybe it's an herb potion you're suspicious of, or a strange exercise regimen guaranteed to make your labor easier. If it seems dangerous, don't do it. Don't worry about giving offense. When it's your (and your baby's) well-being at stake, you can rightfully think about yourself first. Granted, this may feel awkward if it's your mother-in-law enticing you with some traditional ethnic cure that generations of women in her family swear by, but you may as well start somewhere putting up boundaries where your child is concerned.

Always ask your doctor's opinion before undertaking any activity that seems dubious. Put off the advice-giver by saying something vague like, "That sounds interesting. I'll ask my doctor about it on my next visit." Or invoke your doctor's orders if you feel pressured to do something you'd rather not: "My doctor would rather I not try that."

Another shift-the-blame cutoff: "Thanks for your concern, but my doctor says everything's just fine as it is."

Don't Believe Them!

The next time somebody tries to tell you one of these old wives' tales, you can say with perfect sincerity, "You know, I recently read that's just not true."

- Scratching your belly causes stretch marks.
- Cocoa butter or vitamin E lotion prevents stretch marks.
- If you have a lot of heartburn, your baby will have a lot of hair.
- Acne means you're having a girl, because she's "stealing your beauty."
- Lifting your hands over your head will cause the umbilical cord to strangle the fetus.
- Be sure to wear a key during an eclipse to prevent deformities.
- Eating too many strawberries or apples will cause reddish birthmarks.
- Eating spicy foods will burn the baby's eyes.
- Eat what you crave because your body needs that substance (salt, carbohydrate, sugar).
- Now that you're "eating for two" you should double all your portions.
- If you don't indulge your cravings, you'll mark the baby with the shape of the food you denied yourself.
- Walking around barefoot might make the fetus sick.
- If you're frightened by something in pregnancy, your baby will be born with the features or traits of whatever scared you.
- Getting your hair cut during pregnancy robs energy from a growing fetus.
- If you eat fish, your baby will be smarter.
- Don't go swimming or you'll drown the baby.
- If your body hair grows faster than normal during pregnancy, you're carrying a girl.
- If you rub your belly too much, you might make the baby stick to the uterine wall.
- Girls have fast fetal heart rates; boys have slower ones (or vice versa).

- A belly that sticks out mostly in front means it's a boy; carrying all around means it's a girl (or vice versa).
- Carrying high means it's a girl; carrying low means it's a boy (or vice versa).
- Young children can predict the sex of an unborn baby.
- Sex during pregnancy can cause a miscarriage.
- If you don't crave sweets, you must be having a boy.
- Boys cause more morning sickness.
- With every child, your hair gets darker and your teeth get more cavities.
- If a firstborn's first word is "mama," the next child will be a girl; if the firstborn says "dada" first, the next child will be a boy.
- If the woman was more aggressive sexually at conception, the baby will be a boy; if the man was more aggressive, the baby will be a girl.
- A baby conceived in the morning will be a boy.
- Girls cause their mothers' noses to grow larger in pregnancy.
- If you worry too much during pregnancy, your child will be born left-handed.
- Boys are more active in the womb.
- The mother's wedding ring suspended on a string over a pregnant belly can foretell the fetus's sex: If the ring swings back and forth, it's a boy; if it swings in circles, it's a girl.
- You can tell the baby's sex by asking the mother to show you her hands: If she shows them palms up, it's a girl. Palms down, it's a boy.
- Eating spicy foods will trigger labor.
- Having castor oil, mineral oil, olive oil, or a salad with a vinegar dressing will ease a baby's way out the birth canal. (Note: a pregnant woman should only take castor oil under the advice and supervision of her doctor.)

- Walk up stairs, do knee bends, or drive over a bumpy road to induce labor.
- If your mom had a fast labor, you will too.
- Keep newborns indoors for the first week.
- Don't eat fruits or vegetables for the first month after delivery.
- Women with small breasts can't breast-feed.
- Breast-feeding will make your breasts sag.
- Breast-fed babies don't get colic.
- You should bind a quarter or a Band-Aid to your newborn's belly to ensure a firm navel.
- Fat babies always grow into fat children.
- You can't get pregnant while you're breast-feeding.

But These Old Wives' Tales Are True!

Don't automatically rule out advice you hear just because it sounds strange. Some bits of folk wisdom are rooted in good sense. Consider the following truisms:

- **Don't sleep on your back.** Lying flat on your back after the fifth month causes your heavy uterus to compress a major blood vessel, which in turn can decrease blood flow to the fetus. Best of all is to lie on your left side with a pillow between your legs. The right side is okay, too.
- **Drink plenty of water to replenish the waters.** Keeping well hydrated—six to eight eight-ounce glasses of water a day—does indirectly help maintain amniotic

fluid levels. It also reduces constipation, dry skin, and dehydration (which can lead to preterm labor).

- **Stay away from hot tubs or you'll boil the baby.** No, you won't exactly cook your fetus. Excessive heat has been associated with damage to the developing nervous system, though. The first trimester, especially, avoid water temperatures over 102 degrees. This includes Jacuzzis, whirlpools, and hot baths.

- **Pregnancy makes your feet grow.** Blame the presence of hormones that loosen your ligaments (in order to ease the baby through your pelvis at delivery), on top of the thirty or more extra pounds added in a typical pregnancy. Swelling may also play a role. Many women discover their feet grow by a half size or a full size, or a width. Sometimes—but not always—this change is permanent.

- **Nipple stimulation can jump-start labor.** It won't cause labor to begin—no one has yet figured out exactly what triggers the birth process. But stimulation of the nipples can perk up contractions (no pun intended) that have subsided once a woman is already in labor.

- **Second babies are usually easier to deliver.** On average, second labors are shorter than first labors because your cervix and vaginal muscles have already been stretched some. Your pelvic bones may also be wider. *Exception:* If your first delivery was a C-section, the second labor will progress more like a first-timer's.

- **Labor usually starts at night.** The body's production of oxytocin, the hormone that causes contractions, peaks in the evening. Some evolution researchers theorize that this is because humans were designed to give birth at night, when fewer predators were awake.

- **Firstborns are usually late.** The operative word here is "usually," not "always." Just over half of all firstborns are born after their projected due dates, and five percent are born exactly on that date. But 35 percent come before their due dates, making this truism rather meaningless, since you have no way of knowing on which side of the due date your baby will arrive.

UNWANTED ADVICE

What's the best tactic if advice-givers just won't let up?
Persistent pests are the worst kind. They're usually someone very close to you, who abuses that intimacy by crossing the line of good intentions. Instead of advising, they begin haranguing, whether it's about whether to try a vaginal birth after a Cesarean (VBAC) or about the glories of epidurals. Some women do so as a way to validate their own experiences: If they can convert you to their choices, it justifies that they did the right thing, too.

Still, you needn't endure lectures. Instead, cut them off: "Look, it's making me really touchy to talk about this, so let's change the subject." Introduce a new—nonmaternity—topic.

What's the most tactful way to fend off advice from a mother-in-law?
Having a baby often marks a dramatic shift in one's relationship with one's in-laws. Even if you've settled into a wonderful relationship, now there's a very big new thing for her (yes, it's usually the *mother*-in-law) to observe how you

handle. Not only that, it's an arena in which she's well experienced.

Some grandmothers-to-be simply can't help themselves. They view themselves as authorities on babies, and they're itching to share their know-how. The best response is tolerance. Acknowledge her expertise: "I hope we can do as good a job raising our baby as you did with my husband." Make her feel a part of things, whether it's soliciting her advice about layette needs or asking her to share her son's baby book so that you can compare his development with your baby's.

You may find that most of her advice concerns old wives' tales or harmless tips on things like the best way to dress a baby. If it's something you feel very strongly about, though, enlist your partner's support: "Bill and I both feel strongly that breast-feeding is the right thing to do." When the problem escalates, it's imperative that the child of the in-law speak up, too: "Mom, you've got to lay off Susan."

GORY DETAILS

How much detail about prenatal tests is appropriate to discuss?

It depends on your audience. Generally the intimate details of one's health are best left in medical records. Although the results of a triple-screen test or a minute-by-minute description of amniocentesis are fascinating to those people directly involved, they should not be offered up as the subject of conversation at dinner parties, office meetings, or most other social occasions.

But what fun would pregnancy be if we couldn't talk about the pokes and prods undergone at all those doctor visits? That's what girlfriends are for, especially when they are mothers (or better yet, pregnant, too). Comparing notes—in all the biological detail you want—is perfectly fine if you are sure you have a willing ear.

LABOR STORIES

What about those labor-from-hell stories—is there a nice way to say "Shut up"?
Personally, I was as fascinated as dismayed by every anecdote about emergency C-sections, fainting husbands, killer contractions, and women who cursed more than a Quentin Tarantino character in the delivery room. Knowledge is power, after all. Learning about every possible eventuality, whether from a book or a friend, helps prepare you for the reality of labor—maybe not your precise reality, but at least the fact that it's unpredictable and it hurts. I consider this a good thing.

Most storytellers aren't out to scare you. They simply get carried away by the vividness of their own experience. Think of it as a perverse form of motherhood bonding. That said, it's inconsiderate to persist telling stories that are clearly making the listener uncomfortable. So if you've heard enough, change the subject. You don't have to explain yourself, which may only goad on some enthusiastic (or malicious) storytellers. Failing that, you could always excuse yourself and flee to the rest room.

BELLY-RUBBING

Must I let strangers pat my belly?
A big belly *is* magnetic, not to mention pretty hard to ignore. Although it's technically your boundary that's being violated, the offender rarely sees it that way. He (or she, but usually

he) imagines that he is touching the baby. In some cultures, abdominal massage is celebratory.

Before I was expecting, I was dismayed by the idea of a stranger reaching out to touch me. But like many women, I wound up feeling so full of joy and pride that I didn't really mind. I felt like everybody's lucky Buddha. (Except by the ninth month, when I was so full of joy and pride and *baby* that I didn't even want my husband touching me anymore.) It's socially polite to indulge the patter.

Not all women care to tolerate any such intrusion, however, and this is one of your pregnant prerogatives. If you find that you can't stand belly-rubbers, you're well within your Pregnant Woman's Rights to say, "Please stop!" Or say, "Please don't do that, it doesn't feel comfortable." The other person won't know if you're referring to your feelings or your physical state, and no one likes to upset a pregnant woman's physical state.

Some women don't mind family members reaching out to touch them, but are annoyed when perfect strangers do it. Said one such mom: "I've even had people lift my shirt and say, 'Oh, I love bellies!' I just back off, and say, 'Well, sorry but it's attached to the rest of *my* body!' " Another good line: "Look, but don't touch." You could also try patting them back, which is a little bit of tit-for-tat rudeness, not usually advised, but it probably will get your point across!

Do's and Don'ts for Grandparents-to-Be

DO whoop and hug when you hear the news.
DO NOT *squint at the sonogram picture and snort, "Looks like a tadpole to me."*

DO remember that it's your daughter (or daughter-in-law) who's pregnant, not you.
DO NOT *furnish the entire nursery for her as a surprise (at least not without consulting her first).*

DO be supportive about her rabid interest in folic acid, iron, and vitamin B-12.
DO NOT *say, "You know, I drank coffee and smoked Lucky Strikes when I was pregnant, and you turned out okay."*

DO ask her what sorts of things she needs for the baby and offer your expertise pointing out the difference between bassinet sheets, cradle sheets, crib sheets, and pram sheets (and buy as many of them as you please).
DO NOT *throw her a shower. It's not in your job description.*

DO pass along some of your child's own baby pictures or baby books so your son or daughter can compare them with your grandbaby-to-be's.
DO NOT *postpone filling in all the blanks as best you can when your child presents you with one of those "Grandpa's Memories" books, or you'll never get around to it.*

DO say, "Welcome Baby Xavier Khalfani Higgenbottham-Sudzinski!" (or whatever the chosen moniker is) when you first hear the baby's name.
DO NOT *gag, cringe, say, "What's wrong with our names?" or launch a campaign to try to get the parents to change their minds.*

DO offer to help out after the baby arrives, if you can.
DO NOT *assume you'll be welcome to stay for three months.*

DO pitch in and cook some hot meals or run the laundry when you visit.
DO NOT *expect to do nothing but hog the baby and sing lullabies.*

DO present the newborn with a lasting keepsake, whether you make it, had it as a child yourself, or buy it at Tiffany's.
DO NOT *keep asking about it later, as in, "Why do you let her play with that silver rattle? It cost me a bundle!"*

DO pass on your patented, time-tested tips for burping and swaddling.
DO NOT *assume that there has been no progress in child-rearing tactics since you were a new mother.* (**And DO NOT EVER** *turn the baby to sleep on its tummy after your daughter has placed him or her down the correct, safe way, which is on the back or the side.*)

DO tell your son or daughter that he or she makes a wonderful parent.
DO NOT *underestimate how meaningful it will be to hear those words.*

DO pick out a name other than Granny if you prefer it—Mima, Nana, Maisie, Boopsie, Jane, whatever.
DO NOT *go into complete denial that you're becoming grandparent. You are. Get used to it. Love it.*

3

Maternity Clothes

What to wear during your pregnancy is at once intensely private and unavoidably public. It's private because only you know when a waistband or bra that fit fine yesterday suddenly becomes unbearable. Only you know whether Peter Pan collars and polka dots depress you or a pair of leopard-print loafers lifts your spirits. And yet maternity clothes are also constantly seen by others, judged by others—and very often provided by others, too.

Here's what to wear—and how to borrow—with style.

WHEN TO START

When can I start to wear maternity clothes?

Reach for them whenever you feel ready, no matter what anyone else says. For some women, this might mean as early as the second or third month, starting with a pair of forgiving maternity panties or a pretty, loose maternity blouse bought in a burst of proud excitement. Other women are driven by budgetary pinch or disdain for less-than-haute maternity fashions to try making it through to delivery without ever trying on a garment made for pregnant women.

The usual time frame—both from a comfort consideration and in light of how you'll look—is to start using maternity wear around the time you begin to show. You don't want to wait until your front hem is riding two inches higher than your back hem.

No one will fault you for being excited enough to want to dive into maternity shops early on, however. (Beware, you might find those same wonderful clothes getting pretty old by the ninth month.) Nor is there anything wrong with sticking to men's shirts, open jackets, and waistless regular dresses, if your body can handle them. Most women find maternity dressing fun. The selection of clothing today is better than ever. The most practical approach, combining style, comfort, and economy, is to mix specially cut maternity wear with your regular clothes.

BASICS

What's the minimum wardrobe I can get by with?
Your line of work, the climate, and your personal tastes all influence the sort of maternity wardrobe you'll assemble. Perhaps the best-kept secret about maternity clothes is that you don't have to spend a lot of money to look great and to avoid closet boredom in the last trimester.

At a minimum, you'll want two or more comfortable pairs of solid pants (or leggings, if you've got great legs); two tops, preferably tunic length; a dress; and maybe a skirt or shorts, depending on your lifestyle and the weather. Buy these in solid neutral colors (black, navy, white, brown, red) and you've instantly got the versatile backdrop against which you can create dozens of looks. Most women also prefer maternity scaled foundations (bras, panties, hosiery, and possibly a slip) and exercise wear (leotard, swimsuit). A wonderful invention, and a terrific value, are the four-or-more-piece matched sets sold in many maternity shops and department stores, which were pioneered by The Pregnancy Survival Kit from

Belly Basics. They fit, they work together well, they feel stylish, and they allow you to imprint your own "look" on top of them. Add new separates (sweaters, tops, jumpers) as pick-me-ups as your pregnancy progress. If you can sew, there are zillions of maternity patterns, although figuring out which styles look best on you can be a time-consuming process of trial and error.

It's not true, however, that a woman great with child should *only* wear maternity clothes. Pair your maternity basics with blazers and sweaters already in your closet. Borrow vests, cardigans, or long-tailed shirts from your partner. Accessorize with scarves, jewelry, and shoes to complete a look and to create a recognizable version of your usual style. You'll be much happier if your pregnancy style is merely an extension of your customary look rather than if you feel you're masquerading as a kewpie doll.

BORROWING CLOTHES

Would it be all right to ask to borrow a friend's clothes if she's not using them now?
If you're really good friends—the sort who borrow one another's books and party clothes and lawn tools at will—then she'll probably not find you the least bit intrusive to ask.

With everyone else, stick to dropping broad hints: "Well, the baby's not due for five months, and I'm already sick of everything in my closet." Or, "I have no idea what I am going to wear to the Christmas party next week. I don't have any dressy maternity clothes." Then it's up to the friend to volunteer her wardrobe as she chooses.

The reason it's not cool to ask outright is that, technically, her possessions are none of your business. Your friend might secretly be trying to conceive right now. Or the great clothes you remember her wearing during her pregnancy might no longer be in her possession—maybe they were loaners from her sister-in-law, or she donated them to charity. She may not trust you to take proper care of them, though she'd never say as much. Or perhaps she promised them to somebody else.

Most women are only too happy to recycle the maternity outfits that they spent good money on, rather than see them gathering moth holes in the closet. But it's their prerogative to offer, not the pregnant woman's to beg.

Must I wear everything I'm loaned, even clothes that aren't my style?
Don't corner yourself into months of misery like one friend did. When several kind coworkers shared their castoffs, she felt she had to rotate wearing things from each, just to be nice. Unfortunately, one woman's clothes were far fussier than my friend's usual style, another's were quite elegant and made her nervous about spills and snags, and the third had given her some very worn-out things that she felt she needed to also wear, lest the donor take offense. As a result, she spent many days feeling awkward, rather than able to fully revel in her pregnant state.

Maternity dressing is one of the more fun aspects of pregnancy. Try to keep it that way. You're never obligated to wear anything that someone offers you. Few of us are lucky enough to have friends with identical taste, coloring, and bone structures, anyway. Pick your way through loaners and wear only what you love. It's unlikely any affront will be taken. A small maternity wardrobe that you feel good in beats racks of sacks that make you feel like a frump.

What if someone is rude enough to ask why you aren't wearing a certain item? Thank them again for the loan and use one of the following stock answers: "It's so pretty but it didn't fit." "The color isn't me." Or (the catchall), "It just doesn't look right on me yet."

What do I do if I stain a borrowed maternity dress?
When you return the dress, 'fess up and beg forgiveness. But before you rush to replace the item, determine whether the owner will ever use it again. If she's not pregnant or she's through having children, consider making a conciliatory gesture instead. When a dab of spaghetti marred a blouse one woman had borrowed, for example, she included a new scarf with the returned clothes to soften the blow.

If your friend is pregnant again when you return the stained dress, a gift certificate to a maternity store is a nice gesture. Or offer to lend her something of yours. Considering how tired we all get of our maternity wardrobes—didn't your friend seem awfully happy to farm out her clothes to you in the first place?—she may even be secretly thrilled by the need for a nice new replacement the next time she's due.

If a friend gives me some maternity clothes, am I obligated to give them back?
Always establish up front: Is it a gift or a loan? The question is especially pertinent regarding maternity clothes, objects that are useful for only a specific span of time in a woman's life. Many women, once they've finished having kids, couldn't care less what becomes of the clothes. Others are glad to share but might want them back for a future child.

It's the job of the giver to make the distinction clear: "I'm so glad that you can make use of these. Please save them when you're finished, though, because my sister is planning to have a baby soon and I have promised them to her."

Some moms have been known to hang on to borrowed goods with the excuse, "Oh, I got so many things I can't remember what came from whom." If you're the type with a poor memory, write down exactly what each friend lends you.

What's the best way to return borrowed clothes when I'm finished with them?

Always launder or dry-clean anything you borrow and return it in as pristine a state as possible. Fold clothes neatly or hang them in a plastic garment bag.

It's also thoughtful (though not necessary) to give a small thank-you gift when you return the clothes. It could be something as simple as gourmet coffee, a plant, or perhaps a baby item if the woman is expecting again herself.

SHOPPING

Why are maternity-shop clerks so nosy?

The first time you enter a maternity boutique can be exciting—and unnerving, too. I remember slinking into one when I was just a few weeks along, just to scope out the place and see what kinds of clothes I might expect to wear down the line. But I was caught off guard when a perky saleswoman sidled up to me, and purred, "So, when are you due?" In the first place, this seemed like an awfully personal question. And since none of my friends knew about my state yet, I wasn't used to hearing it. I also panicked: If I named my due date, which was still an impossibly distant eight months off, would she laugh?

In fact, salesclerks in maternity shops can be excused for their inquisitiveness. It's assumed that if you're there, you're pregnant. (Although it would be more tactful of them to inquire, "Are you shopping for yourself or for someone else?") Knowing when you're due can help a clerk steer you to the right items: appropriate seasonal choices, styles that can "grow" with you if you're still early on, and so forth. Many shops offer frequent-buyer plans (at the very least you'll probably be buying lots of bras in ever-increasing cup sizes), and they may want to sign you up for one.

If you're just too nervous to admit you're shopping for yourself (and you're not showing yet), simply murmur that you're just browsing or "Thanks but I don't need any help."

DRESSING FOR WORK

Must I wear hose in the office?

From mid-pregnancy on, many pregnant women begin to feel increasingly sausagelike pulling on their hosiery in the morning. If you live in a warm climate or are pregnant in the summer, this fashion convention can become sheer torture. Whether or not to forgo the hose depends on the formality of your office. One rule of thumb: If no one would notice if you went bare in the summer, you can safely do the same when you are pregnant. Fortunately the bare look has become more acceptable, and even fashionable, in recent years.

If you do wear stockings or tights, opt for maternity hose with a high cotton content, which are most comfortable and cut to your expanding proportions. Some women swear by buying larger sizes of their regular brands, but you risk baggy ankles.

If you cannot bear wearing panty hose, try knee-highs with longer skirts (some doctors frown on them, though, because if swelling is a problem for you, they can be binding). Or just say to heck with it and go bare. Your comfort is more important than any fashion convention. Be sure that your shoes are comfortable, however. Especially without hose, the normal foot swelling that can occur late in the day or in hot weather can make favorite pumps and loafers feel like portable pinching prisons. Cornstarch sprinkled inside can help.

What's a professional office look?

Unless, perhaps, you have a very high-profile public position, or are in a conservative profession like banking or law, you don't need to invest in all-new maternity suits and dresses. Most women can safely stick to basic, solid-colored maternity coordinates such as skirts, pants, and dresses, interspersed with their nonmaternity jackets (worn unbuttoned), sweaters, and accent pieces. Don't make the mistake of buying cheap stuff because you'll "only be wearing it for a few months." Better to invest in quality fabrics, since you'll be wearing these garments again and again. Choose things that can stand up to lots of washing and dry cleaning. Supportive undergarments, good shoes, and a great haircut help present a polished look. No matter where you work, leave the "Baby on Board" T-shirt in the closet.

FORMAL DRESSING

What should I wear to a formal party?

Usually the fancier the occasion, the more frantic a woman becomes in trying to find The Perfect Look. Being pregnant can only add to the pressure. *But it doesn't have to!*

To look appropriate at a dressy occasion—whether it's a chic afternoon wedding or a black-tie gala—apply the usual nonpregnant rules of elegant dress. Think simple lines. Think luxurious fabrics. Think wonderful accessories. And to this, I'd add: Don't hide your belly, flaunt it.

You can't go wrong with a basic black dress. Short or long,

it's economical in that it can be worn again in your pregnancy. Choose a clean-lined sheath, A-line, or empire-waist dress. Elegant fabrics such as velvet, brocade, or silk are great if you'll be attending very swanky events; otherwise, even a good stretch cotton in black can be gussied up appropriately. Add fancy earrings and a necklace or pearls. Splurge on dressy shoes. Add a shawl or wrap of sumptuous texture or color, such as satin, pashmina, burned-out velvet, silk, or lace. Don't forget a small dressy handbag in a similar fabric or beaded.

Are form-fitting gowns out during pregnancy?
Not according to the style-setters in Hollywood. Movie starlet moms-to-be accentuate their "bump" all the time in slinky wear that defies any notion that maternity means big and baggy. If you've got a great body—and can find clothes that look made to hug your curves, not merely over-stretched within an inch of propriety—then go for it.

When the Invitation Says...

- *Formal.* Traditionally means men in white tie (white tie, vest, and shirt; black trousers, long tailcoat) and women are in long gowns; true formal affairs are rare, usually swanky evening weddings, and some balls and cotillions.
- *Semi-formal.* Men in black tie (black tuxedo with white shirt) and women in dressy short dresses or long gowns.
- *Black tie.* Same as semiformal.
- *Creative black tie.* Usually indicates a holiday or other theme, where men are expected to wear nontraditional

cummerbunds and vests, or some variation on a costume (as in a theme ball). When in doubt, ask the hostess to clarify.

- *Black tie optional.* Usually means men ought to wear tuxedos but dark business suits are acceptable; women wear cocktail dresses or long, elegant suits in rich fabrics, or the like.
- *Cocktail.* Men in business suits, women in short dresses or in work suits but with dressier accessories.
- *Urban chic.* Newer term denoting upgraded casual wear; not business attire or cocktail-party clothes. Pants and tops are fine for women.
- *Casual* or *informal.* Let the event and your hostess be your guide.

CASUAL DRESSING

Can a pregnant woman wear a bikini?

If a pregnant woman thinks she can, then more power to her! It helps, of course, to have started the pregnancy with a toned body that looked great in that style. While many sunbathers are unaccustomed to the sight in our relatively buttoned-up country, a pregnant woman in a bikini is neither tasteless nor inappropriate. (I've seen more flesh on some men's midriffs at the beach.) The suit should fit comfortably over her derrière. For added comfort, look for maternity tankini (longer top, bikini bottom) styles or two-piece suits with matching cover-ups.

POST-BABY

Can I wear maternity clothes after the baby's born, if I need to?
You'll probably need to, at least for a little while. The truth is that nobody leaves the hospital carrying a newborn while wearing her prematernity blue jeans. For some weeks afterward, while their bodies realign and they shed the weight accumulated during pregnancy, most new moms must wear the same clothes they did during mid-pregnancy (at about four to six months along). Breast-feeding can further limit wardrobe choices, because your bust may be larger than it was prepregnancy, and you'll want tops with easy-access. (So long to those maternity dresses, unless they have buttonfronts.) Think function before fashion—for just a little bit longer.

Comfortable postpartum choices include:

- maternity pants or leggings
- pants or leggings with elastic waistbands or drawstring waists
- elastic-waistband skirts (or maternity skirts)
- maternity tops (the ones that aren't voluminous)
- button-front shirts
- nursing tops or dresses (especially designed for breast-feeding, they have discreet openings)
- oversize T-shirts

4

Tricky Issues

*I*n some ways, being pregnant is like attending a state dinner at the White House or visiting India for the first time. If you've never experienced it before, how are you supposed to know how to act in the many new situations that you encounter along the way? It's a whole new world out there now.

Consider the following advice on how to navigate the trickier moments of pregnancy.

REST ROOMS

How should I handle my exit when I have to get to a bathroom in a hurry?
Quickly and quietly. If you can get the words out, "Excuse me," will do. There's no need to say where you're headed, much less why.

Can I cut ahead in long ladies' room lines if I need to?
Some pregnant women go so far as to avoid concerts, the theater, shopping malls at Christmas, and other locations where too many women must simultaneously converge on too few bathroom stalls. But pregnant women need those change-of-pace outings, so enjoy them.

Don't abuse the privilege, but if you really can't make it

through a long line, no one should fault you for speaking up. Certainly no woman who's ever carried around her own pregnant bladder would, and in a long line there are bound to be several such compatriots.

Expectant mothers who are showing have the easiest time breaking queues. (It helps to wear outfits that accentuate your belly on such outings.) All you need to say is, "Excuse me, please, but do you mind if I cut in? It's really an emergency." If you're not showing, add, "I'm pregnant." Look grateful and say thanks when you get the go-ahead.

NAUSEA

What do I do if I get sick in public?
Morning sickness is worst for the majority of expectant mothers during the first twelve weeks. Rest assured that most of the time, you'll get to a rest room in time. But when accidents occur, dole out profuse apologies once you recover, and clean up after yourself. Immediately offer to pay for the professional cleaning of a rug, chair, pillow, or whatever was soiled. If your hostess demurs, find out what it would cost to clean such an item and send a check. If you're at your workplace and public (rather than private) property has been damaged, this gesture is not necessary as a cleaning service is probably regularly employed.

You'll probably feel mortified but don't beat yourself up over it. People will forgive and soon forget.

Needless to say, one should make every effort to reach a bathroom or at least to get outdoors. As soon as you arrive in a new place, map out potential exits. If possible, learn to recognize what triggers your nausea (certain smells, for example) so you can be forewarned. If you suffer severe morning sickness, discreetly carry a bandanna or handkerchief during the first trimester. Sound too old-fashioned? Think of it as funkily stylish. Besides, it's more durable than a Kleenex tissue.

DOCTOR'S APPOINTMENTS

What can I do if my doctor always leaves me waiting forever?
It was irksome enough when you had to squander two hours once a year just waiting for a Pap smear. When you're visiting your obstetrician monthly—or more often, later in pregnancy—lengthy waits can become truly annoying. Most ob-gyns organize their schedules to maximize patient flow. But the best-run offices can't foresee an emergency C-section or other problem that causes delays. A certain degree of waiting is just part of the experience. To make use of the time, bring a good pregnancy guide with you (or the latest *National Enquirer*), or catch up on work.

If long waits are a chronic problem, address it directly to your doctor. Ask why this is the case. You're a customer, after all, and deserve respect. If you don't have time to waste, maybe you need to make a switch in your prenatal care. Consider moving to a practice with a larger number of physicians, who tend to rotate their shifts so that someone is always available for appointments while someone else is handling emergencies or deliveries. Also try to schedule early-morning appointments, which tend to be less affected by backups and delays.

What should I do if I feel my doctor rushes me?
Refuse to be intimidated. Come to your appointments with a prepared list of questions, no matter how trivial they may seem. (There are no "dumb" questions when you're preg-

nant.) This will prevent your blanking in the rush of the moment. Insist on going down the list and receiving a satisfactory answer to each question. Ask follow-ups. If you still don't understand, be persistent. Say, "I know you may see this problem everyday, but it's my first pregnancy. Can you explain it again?" If your doctor waves you off or continually gives more vague explanations than you prefer, perhaps you need a new physician.

Don't be afraid to address the situation directly: "I'm feeling like you're hurrying me, Doctor. Is there something more important than me that you've got to do?" If he or she says yes, that's the wrong answer. Nothing should be more important to a caregiver than the woman dangling her legs on his or her exam table right at the moment.

How do I proceed if I really like my doctor, as a person, and want to be friends?

A unique relationship is forged with one's caregiver during the nine months of pregnancy. The doctor knows all about your life, you might learn a bit about his or hers. You've frankly discussed such personal matters as your hopes and fears about your baby. Watching this person in action, it's natural to respect and admire their professional qualities as well as personal traits. Certainly you see each other regularly enough.

It's easy to mistake these natural warm feelings for personal attraction. Some women even experience a sort of mourning for their doctor, once the baby is delivered and those frequent checkups are a thing of the past. Should you invite him or her out to lunch? To your next party?

Despite the very intimate nature of something so emotional as bringing a new life into the world, the pregnant woman must always remember this: Your relationship with your obstetrician is a professional one, not a personal one.

If you meet again and befriend one another outside of the clinic or hospital, that's one thing. But otherwise, stick to saying hello during your annual exams and sending photos of your baby to adorn the office walls.

SWITCHING HEALTH PROFESSIONALS

How do I tell a friend I don't like the doctor or childbirth educator she's recommended?
Speak the truth. Many preferences and prejudices enter into the selection of a doctor, midwife, or other childbirth professional. It's smart to network through friends for recommendations. Ultimately, though, whom you choose to work with is a personal matter.

Thank your friend for her suggestion and, while avoiding insulting her, simply give the reason you plan to consult an alternative: "I know Dr. X has a great reputation, but I think I'd prefer someone who can spend a bit more time with patients." Or, "Thanks for recommending Sue Blue for Lamaze class. I enjoyed meeting her. But I think I want to take classes from someone who's more supportive about natural childbirth than she seems to be."

I trust my doctor but I don't really *like* her—does this matter?
Yes. You may have chosen your doctor based on the quality of care he or she provides, but if you don't feel comfortable with that person, it can be a hindrance to your treatment. Pregnancy is such an emotional time already, it doesn't make sense to layer on unnecessary simmering resentment, anger, or discomfort. As a result, you may wind up not providing the most helpful answers to certain questions. Or your personal dislike may lead you to mistrust the answers your doctor

gives you, or to not take his or her recommendations seriously enough. Don't worry about hurting the professional's feelings (see the next question). If you don't click, make the switch as early as possible in your pregnancy.

What's the polite way to switch obstetricians?

Assuming you haven't moved to a new city, most women go looking for a new health caregiver because they aren't happy with their current choice. Whatever you do, don't stick with a doctor whose manner or policies you dislike for fear of being rude or out of a reluctance to rock the boat.

The doctor-patient relationship is, ultimately, a business partnership. It's perfectly appropriate to fire your old doc and hire a new one without a word of explanation. On the other hand, your doctor (and indirectly, other patients in the practice) can benefit from hearing the cause of your discontent. Mention it when you write to request the timely transfer of your medical records to your new prenatal caregiver.

How do I switch childbirth-preparation classes if I don't like my first choice?

Do let your instructor know if you plan to leave the class because the location or time is inconvenient. She will also appreciate knowing if the content is simply not what you were hoping for. For example, some couples sign up for the Bradley Method, only to decide they prefer something less intense. (Bradley advocates husband-coached childbirth and the avoidance of all drugs, emphasizes nutrition and exercise, and requires many outside readings.) Or a hospital-based class may focus too narrowly on the procedures recommended at that institution (use of IV or laboring in bed, for example), but the couple wants to hear about a broader range of possibilities.

The very best courses are taught by an independent instructor, meeting for an hour or two each session over a period of several weeks. All-in-one-day sessions cover too much material to be adequately absorbed in one sitting. It's wise to read up in advance on the various childbirth methods (such as Bradley, Lamaze, or Read) and to find out a bit about the instructor's orientation. That way, you're not caught unawares at the first class.

Sometimes the instructor's personality clashes with the pregnant woman's or her partner's. There may be something that you simply don't like about her. Because the information and techniques she's imparting are so important, it's worthwhile to mesh well with the teacher. If you don't wish to continue classes with her, it's not necessary to give this reason. Simply switch to another class.

Caution: Before leaving a class, get signed up for a replacement one that can be completed well before your due date. Some childbirth classes have waiting lists or do not admit newcomers once they've started a session. It's smart timing to begin childbirth classes in the seventh month and plan to finish either late in the eighth month or early in the ninth.

FINDING OUT THE BABY'S SEX

Should we, or shouldn't we?
Whether or not you find out the baby's gender before birth is strictly a matter of personal taste. My husband and I, for example, relished the grand mystery of not knowing. It was a big surprise to look forward to at the end of nine months. (But then, I'm not the type who roots around for her Christmas presents or who reads ahead to the last page of a novel, either.) More seriously, not knowing whether I was carrying

a boy or a girl helped me from getting too attached, in the terrible, unlikely event something went wrong.

Certainly the temptation to learn the baby's gender is strong, considering the availability of prenatal testing. Some factors to consider:

Why parents like to find out:

- They can prepare a gender-specific nursery
- They only have to agree on one name
- They can buy pink or blue clothes
- They prefer to know everything possible about the fetus
- Because medical advances have made knowing the gender possible, why not?

Why parents don't like to find out:

- It's not what nature intended
- They want a big surprise to look forward to
- They don't want to start sex-stereotyping their child even before birth
- They get to choose two names
- They don't want to be stunned if the ultrasound turns out to be wrong! (This happens more often than you might think.)

My husband wants to know the baby's gender but I don't— who should concede?

Since the mother is the one in whose body the baby resides, it ultimately should be her decision whether to discover the baby's gender. A loving partner should respect her decision— even if he holds the opposite viewpoint.

On the other hand, if the mother chooses to find out, but the father doesn't want to know, it's equally uncaring of her to run out and paint the nursery pink or blue. Likewise, it's not fair for a father-to-be to cross-examine the ultrasound attendant or to peek at amniocentesis records, if they've previously agreed not to find out. (My brother-in-law actually did the former. Bless his heart, he kept the secret from my sister for several months, until she became consumed by the inequity of his knowing and her not, and begged him to tell her, which he did, in poetry, as her Mother's Day present.)

Whatever you decide, realize that this is just one of the first of many many instances in which, as parents, you'll have to arrive at a consensus.

What do we do if the ultrasound technician teases us that she can tell the baby's sex and we don't want to know—or worse, she actually spills the beans?

Unexpected things can happen when the magical image of your baby's white pulsing heart appears on the monitor screen. One couple vowed they wouldn't find out, only to be tempted at the last minute by a technician who blurted out, in a singsong voice, "I know what it is!"

"Okay, tell us!" they begged. Later, the sheepish mom said she felt like she'd snarfed a whole bag of chocolate at one sitting or opened all her birthday presents early. On the other hand, another woman was gleeful to have learned this information by accident.

Whatever happens ought to be your choice, no one else's. Your decision about whether to find out is yours alone, period. Health-care practitioners who fail to respect your wishes ought to have a sonogram of their heads (and hearts) taken to see if anything's in there. At the very least, such spoilsports ought to be reported to your supervising obstetrician. They broke a social contract with you, and by reporting them, you may be able to spare future couples the same disappointment.

Try to prevent unexpected news by making your wishes

clear in a very serious tone before an ultrasound begins. Remind the technician: "We'd like you to follow a don't-ask, don't-tell policy about the baby's sex. We are not going to ask you because we don't want to know, so please don't tell us." Sometimes the sex is obvious in a spread-legged fetus, but you may be marveling too much at the very sight of your baby to notice unless this is pointed out. (Even high-tech sonograms can be hard for the layperson to read.) A respectful doctor or nurse will avoid, or not linger, on the telltale parts.

Anyone having an ultrasound should remember that this is not a foolproof method for determining the fetus's gender. Many an umbilical cord has been misread as a penis.

If you've had amniocentesis, or CVS, take care flipping through your patient files. The baby's gender will usually be cited in the report. Some doctors avoid slips of the tongue by making it a point to refer to all fetuses as "him" or "her" and telling parents this in advance.

IN TRANSIT

May I ask someone to give up their seat for me on the subway or bus?
It used to be that women were always given a seat by the men around them. Now not even elderly women, much less pregnant women, are afforded this courtesy. Some say, if a woman can hold the same job as a man, why can't she stand up on the subway like a man? And this is generally considered fair enough these days—all other things being equal.

But men don't get pregnant. They have no idea what it's like to stand for long minutes on swollen ankles and too tight shoes, lurching on the train while a little life-form inside is performing its own somersaults. Any young, healthy man (or nonpregnant woman, for that matter) who sits without offering a seat while in view of an obviously pregnant woman, particularly on a long commute, deserves to suffer six months of morning sickness.

Rather than putting yourself at the mercy of others' kindness, be proactive yourself. Ask for a seat, if you need one.

Can I use a handicapped-parking spot when I'm pregnant?
By the last month of pregnancy, when waddling great distances gets tough, many moms-to-be could certainly use the convenience of a close-in parking spot. The trouble with using the designated handicapped spot is that most areas fine drivers who park cars not bearing a Handicapped Parking license plate, windshield sticker, or rearview mirror hanger.

Some shops aim to get around this inconvenience by designating special "stork spots" for pregnant customers. There's also a movement under way to help pregnant women obtain temporary handicapped-parking passes through their ob-gyn office for use during the last month. Although such conveniences are for women who are pregnant, this doesn't mean you're entitled to use them simply because two lines showed up on your pregnancy test. If you're otherwise in good health, park farther back and walk until you're late in your eighth month. (Hey, it's good exercise.)

Can I use a pregnancy-parking spot after my baby is born?
Definitely yes. This is their intention, to be used both during late pregnancy and in the neonatal period, for about the first four to six weeks. Thus the usual name, "stork spots." That time period is when the mother is still recuperating and getting used to lugging a car seat with a slumbering newborn.

How can I avoid unnecessary hassles when traveling?
Here are the Pregnant Woman's Rules for Travel, which

are guaranteed to make trips better for you and those around you:

- *Go somewhere!* Ideally, on a romantic escape. Soon enough, getting away will be complicated by having to hire a sitter, pump breast milk, and tear yourself away from your beloved bambino. In other words, you may not want to go anywhere for months and months. Go now and make yourself—and your partner—very happy.
- *But go at the right time.* Roughly months four through seven are best. Travel in the first trimester is often ruined by morning sickness and overwhelming fatigue. (I once went ahead with a preplanned cross-country skiing trip in Montana and spent most of it on the bed in my cabin.) The risk of miscarriage also makes overseas travel ill advised in early pregnancy. You don't want to risk hemorrhaging on a long flight or undergoing a D&C in a strange hospital where you may not even speak your doctor's language. By the eighth month, you may feel too uncomfortable for big trips, and in the ninth month you'll be advised to stick close to home in case you go into labor. Often airlines and cruise lines refuse to board passengers late in their pregnancies without a doctor's written okay.
- *Book an aisle seat.* By plane or train, you don't want to have to lumber over your fellow passengers on your repeated visits to the rest room. An aisle seat is also convenient because you ought to get up and stretch your legs periodically.
- *Bring along your own water.* Not only will you and your happily hydrated fetus be grateful, but also you'll spare the flight attendant from making constant extra trips over to you for refills.

- *Build in extra time on road trips.* You may be making one pit stop an hour, or more. Factor this in when you tell someone your expected arrival time to spare them unnecessary worry.
- *Pack light.* You may have to tote your own bags, even for a short distance, which can be cumbersome when your center of gravity is displaced. Even if you don't carry your own, it's nice to spare others the trauma of an overloaded case. You'll also save yourself minutes of fussing over which outfit to put on, when you should be enjoying every last minute of traveling without a baby in tow.
- *Wear comfortable shoes.* Factor in water retention (which can cause swelling) and long schleps down airport terminals or city streets. One-to-two-inch heels are both safe and supportive.

Great Escapes

Be nice to your partner—and yourself—and go somewhere during pregnancy. Go someplace by yourselves, and preferably somewhere that does not cater to kids. (You'll see enough of Disney World in a few years.) Some nice ideas:

- A romantic country inn
- A swanky suite at a fine hotel
- A condo on the beach—not during school breaks
- The place you honeymooned
- An all-inclusive resort
- A cabin in the woods

- A cruise
- A B&B in a big city

SMOKERS

How should I ask a smoker at the next table in a restaurant to refrain?
Fortunately nonsmoking sections are the norm, rather than the exception these days. (And, of course, in many cities no smoking is permitted in any restaurant or bar.) But if you have the misfortune to be seated somewhere smoke can find you, you should first ask the server if you can be moved to a less offensive place.

If this is not possible, muster your courage to confront the offender: "Excuse me, but would you mind putting out your cigarette? I'm afraid there are no other tables available, and the smoke is not very healthy for me because I'm pregnant." If the person is considerate, they'll agree. Be prepared for the possibility, however, that your concern for your baby's health will be met with rudeness. If the smoker persists, you must choose between suffering in silence (and both your pride and your fetus will suffer) or finding a more hospitable place to eat, with a more pleasing air.

COMPLAINTS

How much am I entitled to complain without stepping over the line into rudeness?
Complaints are no fun for listeners, whether the complainer is sick, tired, pregnant, or all three. That said, there is plenty to complain about over the average nine months of preg-

nancy. The stomach-churning smell of sausage frying, the long walk from your car to your office, adolescent-style acne, lengthy doctor waits—take your pick. Just because you're expecting doesn't mean you have to be a beatific madonna all the time. Even the unflappable Melanie Wilkes moaned a little during her pregnancy scenes in *Gone With the Wind*.

Very good friends (and very good mates) will endure a certain amount of complaining because it's part of their job description. Just be careful not to abuse their love. Cues you've overdone it:

- More than half of your conversation begins with "I"
- Your companion is staring off into the middle distance
- The sympathetic smile on his or her face begins to look forced, especially if accompanied by glazed eyes

Every pregnant woman ought to have some outlets for her turbulent emotions besides her partner. A friend who's at a similar stage of pregnancy is ideal, assuming either of you can get a word in edgewise. A journal is also a great way to vent.

Complaints to strangers—particularly complaints that are intimate in nature, as many pregnancy woes are—ought to be kept to a minimum.

One kind of complaint that's perfectly correct is a polite protest regarding poor service or otherwise uncomfortable conditions. Feel free to speak up if, for example, someone is smoking in a nonsmoking area of a restaurant, or your fish is cooked insufficiently (both of which are health hazards during pregnancy, and none too appetizing at other times, either).

SOCIAL OBLIGATIONS

Is it appropriate to agree to be a bridesmaid in a wedding if you're pregnant?
Yes. The social taboo against participating in public events while great with child has disappeared. (Heck, even pregnant brides have become so commonplace that some bridal shops keep special maternity wedding gowns in their regular stock. But that's more a matter of morality than manners.)

A bride should choose her bridesmaids based on her relationships with them, not on whether they can fit into a pink size-6 taffeta gown. Of course, the woman who is pregnant should agree only if she feels physically able. If the would-be bridesmaid's due date is within a few weeks of the wedding date, it might be prudent to excuse herself. And both bride and bridesmaid should be open-minded about the fact that anything can happen during pregnancy. Circumstances such as prescribed bed rest or premature labor may prevent the mom-to-be from making it to the altar.

Is it okay to ask a bridesmaid to drop out of one's wedding if she becomes pregnant during the planning phase?
See the above answer. Friendship makes the bridesmaid, not her appearance. To kick someone off a wedding party because her big belly might spoil the symmetry of the wedding photos is pretty low. A gown can always be altered. (The bridesmaid should foot the cost.) Exception: If the bridesmaid is unmarried and the bride has a strong moral objection, that's a different matter, since a wedding is a religious ceremony. The would-be bridesmaid should excuse herself if she senses a potential conflict.

BED REST

What's the best way to solicit friends' help if I'm on bed rest?
Ask for help, and in as specific a way as possible. The good friends you're most likely to enlist probably already are wondering what they can do for you. Up to 20 percent of expectant moms wind up spending a week or more in bed. The degree of bed rest that's prescribed can vary. Some women are not allowed to so much as move in bed, while others can sit up and eat or even take a shower, though they may not leave the house. Your friends are apt to have many questions about the sort of help you most need. Housecleaning? Grocery runs? Errands to get the nursery ready? Renting videos? Minding an older child? Simple companionship for those long dull days of waiting? Do you have one-time tasks they can perform, or are there some things that would be helpful on an ongoing basis?

Whatever you do, don't be shy. Your baby's health depends on the kindness of others, so that you can properly follow doctor's orders. If someone calls to offer assistance, accept it graciously: "Yes, I'd love it if you would come by and bring me some new magazines. Just seeing you would lift my spirits." You're doing them a favor in accepting their civility.

After your baby has been born and you're back on your feet, host a lunch for the friends who helped you through those difficult weeks.

Am I supposed to dress nicely if I'm on bed rest or should visitors expect to find me in my pajamas?
Never mind about visitors' expectations. Your main objective on bed rest is to preserve your baby's health, decorum be

darned. You're apt to feel better, though, if you indulge in your favorite pick-me-up rituals. For example, use a little makeup, shave your legs, or exchange your pajamas for a nice maternity tunic and clean leggings. If you're the loungewear type, consider sending someone to buy you a pretty bed jacket, an old-timey indulgence that's worth the cost-per-wear if you're stuck in bed day after day.

If you refuse to succumb to slothdom, you'll feel better mentally and be more enjoyable to be around.

Could I ask a hairdresser to come cut my hair at home if I'm on bed rest?
Feel-good routines boost a bedridden mom-to-be's spirits enormously. Many stylists will make house calls for their loyal customers. So might manicurists and masseuses. All you need to do is ask. Add another 5 to 10 percent to your customary tip.

What can I say if people try to get me to get out of bed?
Sometimes partners, relatives, and others on whom the burden falls when a mom-to-be must be bed-bound begin to question whether the precaution is all that necessary. It may seem like the mom is "just lying around" while they have so much to do. Surely, they may rationalize, that a little activity can't hurt.

Bed rest is hard on relationships. This is especially true if the mother's income is reduced as a result. But it's wisest to follow doctor's orders—not Daddy's or your mom's. Get a second opinion if you're doubtful.

Tell the person that you need their support to comply with doctor's orders. Complaints only make it harder, and put your baby at risk. Another good idea: Have your partner or other scoffing relatives tour a neonatal intensive-care unit. There they can witness the very real perils of a baby who is born too soon.

MISCARRIAGE

What should be done in the event of a miscarriage?
The bereaved parents need not say or do anything. Their own immediate family will learn what has happened and they can quietly spread the word among family and friends as necessary.

Friends should let the family mourn as they prefer. Some couples need some time in seclusion while others find it helpful to gather their nearest and dearest around them. Express your sadness for them. It's fine to inquire if there is anything you can do to help. (For example, there may be people the parents would like a friend to inform. Or in the event of a late miscarriage or a stillbirth, the mother may later ask to have her shower gifts returned.)

Neutral condolences are often best: "We're so sorry to hear of your loss." "We share your grief." "Please know what you are in our thoughts and prayers."

It is *not* helpful to say:

- "It's probably for the best."
- "It's God's will."
- "If only you hadn't worked so hard/exercised so much/ kept on smoking," etc.
- "At least it wasn't a real baby yet."
- "At least it was here too brief a time for you to become really attached."
- "It's not like you lost an older child."
- "You're still so young. You have plenty of time for parenthood."
- "Don't worry, you can get pregnant again soon."

APRÉS-BABY HELPERS

How do we break it to my mother and my mother-in-law, who live out of town, that we don't want them to come help us after the baby is born?
Before you make any hasty decisions, consider their motivations and whether you have other resources for assistance in their place. In their favor, the new grandmothers have much more experience with children than the new parents do. They've been there. So above all, be open-minded.

While pregnant with my firstborn, I was fairly adamant that I wouldn't want company. Then my mother suggested that she and my father, along with my ninety-year-old grandmother, drive the six hundred miles to my home to arrive the day the baby and I were discharged from the hospital. (He was their first grandchild and great-grandchild, respectively.) My dad and my gram would stay a few days and then leave my mother with us for three weeks.

I was apprehensive. I envisioned my husband, our cooing bundle, and me all cuddled together spinning our own new-family bonds, insulated from the realities of the world in a cottony bright, laundry-detergent-commercial sort of fantasy. In reality, however, life with a new baby is full of chaos, fatigue, and leaking body fluids. Complicating matters for me, my son was born ten days early the day before his father was to start law school.

As it turned out, I couldn't wait to show off the baby to these beloved visitors. They were waiting in the driveway when we got back from the hospital. My dad ran errands. My gram held the baby and looked tickled pink. And my mom cooked, made ice packs to soothe my red-hot, milk-filling breasts; fielded the phone; stayed up half the night with me for feedings; and helped me get to doctor's checkups (of which there were many, as my son had jaundice and needed repeated blood tests). When she left three weeks later, I waved good-bye from the driveway with tears streaming down my face.

Mothers (and mothers-in-law) know firsthand that new moms need help. That they also get to meet their brand-new grandchild is icing on the cake. Even if the new father has paternity leave from work, an extra set of experienced hands can be very welcome. Or you could arrange your mother's visit to begin as soon as Daddy's leave ends. Mothers, by the way, deserve first dibs over mothers-in-law, since it's their flesh and blood who just gave birth.

Of course, not all parents make great helpers. If your parents are the type who generally require a great deal of fuss and entertaining when they visit, consider setting some kindly ground rules in advance: "You know I will be keeping to bed for the first week, and we can't take you anywhere. But we'd love to have you stay from Saturday through Tuesday and meet the baby." Or you could make arrangements for out-of-towners to stay at a local hotel.

What if you know your parents too well and even this much interaction will only set you up for meddling and make-work? Then head them off at the pass. Say something like, "I know you might be hoping to stay with us after the baby is born, but things will be so chaotic that we think it would be best if we came to see you for Thanksgiving instead. You know Bill has a few weeks off from work to help me out, and Sue has promised to check in every day." Be firm: "This is what I really want."

WATER BREAKING

What should I do if my water breaks on someone else's rug?
Rest assured that every pregnant woman's nightmare is rarely

a reality. Only about one in ten women's membrane ruptures before labor begins. Even then, it typically occurs in the calm of evening, and it may be just a trickle. Still, it helps to have a game plan throughout the third trimester. If you're worried about the possibility of your water breaking at work, designate a colleague as point person to whisk you off to privacy (or the hospital). If it happens on the street, get help. This is no time to be shy or self-conscious about the wet stain on your skirt. Get a towel, as you'll continue to leak.

And if the unthinkable happens in the middle of a meeting or a cocktail party? Humor is a great way to deal with awkward moments. Suggests Jeanne Martinet, author of *The Faux Pas Survival Guide*, "After that huge, horrid pause that follows you could say something like, 'I *hate* when that happens!' or 'Don't worry—I'm just marking my territory.' " Then again, you may be too astonished for a quick quip.

Don't worry about cleanup—it's more important that you alert your doctor pronto. After the baby's born you should offer to pick up the cleaning tab (though the odds are good you'll be refused).

GUARDIANS

How do we tell friends or family that we've picked someone else to be our child's guardian?
Who will be your child's legal guardian(s) in the event of your premature demise is a private matter. An announcement not expected. So don't feel obligated to issue one. Still, this can be a dicey matter, since relatives are the ones most apt to inquire, and to take offense if they are not chosen. Should someone ask whom you've picked, it's best simply to give the names. You don't have to explain why, other than, "We thought it was for the best."

Do's and Don'ts for Best Friends

DO express only gladness and excitement when she tells you the news.
DO NOT *sound disappointed because you've just lost another one to The Other Side.*

DO be empathetic when she describes her travails in trying to locate a size 40EEE bra.
DO NOT *say, "Well if you think your breasts are sore now, wait until you start nursing!"*

DO lend her your best old maternity clothes.
DO NOT *insist that she come and see you model the form fitting, size-6 designer tube dress you just bought.*

DO keep sharing good gossip with her, even if it's hard to get a word in edgewise with her endless pregnancy talk.
DO NOT *shout out, "That's it! Not another word about morning sickness, prenatal tests, baby names, and Laura Ashley Mother & Child wallpapers!"*

DO gently remind her to keep up with those Kegels (she'll thank you later).
DO NOT *share tales of thirty-six-hour labors and yard-long epidural needles that just wouldn't stay in unless she's really begging you to tell them.*

DO gently speak up when she's about to drive right past your exit in an absentminded fog.

DO NOT *crack jokes about whether or not she can fit behind the steering wheel anymore.*

DO offer your opinions on the relative merits of Winnie the Pooh versus Paddington Bear.
DO NOT *say "Why bother decorating a nursery? You'll just have to do it all over again in five years when the baby grows into a kindergartner."*

DO offer to host her shower and solicit her input on whom to invite and whether or not she really wants to play Can You Identify the Baby Slop?
DO NOT *enclose her gift wish list in your invitations, although you may cheerfully pass on such information on the phone, provided the other guests request it first.*

DO help her organize a brigade of cooks, cleaning help, and errand-runners if she must be bedridden for a spell.
DO NOT *ask her if she minds keeping an eye on your two-year-old while you run out to the store since she's just lying around the house anyway.*

DO tell her to call you when the baby's born, no matter what time it is.
DO NOT *groggily say "A boy? Terrific. Let me buzz you back later," when the proud new parents call at 3 A.M.*

DO tell her that the new baby is adorable and looks just like her.
DO NOT *add, "Well not as adorable as my little Junior, of course."*

5

At Work

It's been said that the workplace is like a second family. We often see our colleagues more than our own relatives. We get to know their personalities, quirks, and habits. So when one of the gang is pregnant, everyone notices. And comments. And reacts. Or wonders how to act.

Despite the collegiality of many workplaces, and the fact that pregnancy is such an intimate experience, the workplace is ultimately a place ruled by a professional code of conduct. (This is true even if it's a casual, zany, fun sort of office.) No matter how excited you are, no matter how happy everyone is for you, at the end of the day, the work must get done.

The following considerations balance the formal and the familiar of office politics for the parent-to-be.

TELLING OTHERS

Must I disclose my pregnancy to prospective employers while interviewing for a job?
The law is on your side. According to the Federal Pregnancy Discrimination Act, companies of a certain size are forbidden to discriminate against hiring a pregnant woman as long as she can do the job. You are not obligated, however, to dis-

close your pregnancy up front. What matters most are your qualifications.

That said, it's courteous to inform your interviewer at some point—perhaps after an offer is made. Legally, she can't retract the offer, and your honesty can set a positive tone for your working relationship. The employer may need to make plans now for your eventual temporary absence. There are always mitigating circumstances to weigh, though. Ultimately it's your call.

When should I tell my colleagues that I'm pregnant?

There you are, bursting with enthusiasm. You've already told your family and your closest friends. So it's natural to want to tell the people who see you most often—your coworkers. Before you blurt the words, however, think twice. It's usually not a good idea to spread word of your pregnancy throughout the workplace as soon as you know.

The first colleague to hear the news ought to be your immediate supervisor. You don't want rumors to precede the facts. The word always ought to come directly from you, who can put the brightest, most reassuring spin on the news. But don't rush into the boss's office the first day you know. It's usually best if you hold off telling until the third or fourth month, when you begin to show.

Exception: You have good reason to inform your supervisor of your pregnancy right away if you work in hazardous conditions. Examples: with chemicals or cleaning solvents, in a place where you are exposed to viruses or x rays, or in a job that requires a lot of standing or physical exertion. Don't delay out of fear of disrupting the work routine. Your baby's health is paramount, and the first trimester is a particularly critical time to shield your developing fetus. You might also want to time your announcement on the early side if you work in a cyclical job, such as in retail or education, where it would benefit your employer to have advance notice to find someone who'll cover for you.

Without a good reason to announce a pregnancy prematurely, it's merely unproductive. Even after the first flurry of congratulations, your condition will persist in serving as a magnet for conversation, which will soon get tiresome. "Do you think you can stay awake through this meeting?" "Gee, you've been pregnant an awfully long time." "Wow, you look huge today." Colleagues may think differently of you, possibly to your detriment when it comes to handing out assignments or conducting future planning. Finally, because the odds of miscarriage are highest during the first three months, you risk making a personal tragedy into a public event should you tell too soon.

What's the best way to inform my boss?
Whether you say it straight or do so humorously is a question of style. (One woman ordered pickles and ice cream while out to lunch with her supervisor.) Your approach depends a lot on the personalities of both your workplace and your boss. However you say it, you must be professional, positive, and prepared.

Tell your supervisor in a private meeting, not in front of others. Consider scheduling it for a Friday afternoon, so that your boss has the weekend to absorb the news. People tend to be in a better mood then, too. Realize that he or she may be happy for you, but understandably nervous about how your absence, whether temporary or permanent, will affect business.

Be upbeat. If you couch the news in tentative or worried tones, your supervisor is apt to mirror them. But if you're happy and confident, you'll be reassuring. Frame your words in terms of your proven value to the company: "While being pregnant is very exciting to me, you don't need to worry about it being a distraction to my work. I've been a top performer for three years in this department and I don't expect that to change."

Finally, and most importantly, think through an action plan. No, you don't need to have everything figured out yet. You should, however, be able to make some suggestions to your boss about approximately how long you plan to work (up to the last minute? Until a predetermined date?) and how much leave you intend to take. Do some advance planning. Contact your human-resources representative to find out how much leave, both paid and unpaid, you are eligible for. (He or she is required to keep your confidence.) Factor in vacation time, too. Also investigate what sorts of family-friendly options are available at your firm: Flextime? Part-time schedules? Working from home? What have other colleagues done? Finding out about options and precedents helps you and your supervisor make the best possible plans.

Also give some thought to how your work will be handled in your absence. Can parts of it be doled out among different people? Will you need to train a replacement? Can you make suggestions as to who the best candidates might be? What about workload—are there certain projects you can move up to complete now, or others you can postpone?

Don't try to hash out all the details at your initial meeting with your supervisor. Say, "If you agree, I'd like to take a couple weeks to sort out an action plan and then get back together to discuss what needs to happen before I leave." This gives your supervisor a chance to mull the options, too. Then arrange a later meeting at which you can discuss how your workload will be handled in your absence, who needs special briefings on your work, and so on.

MATERNITY LEAVE

What preparations should I make in advance of my departure?
Start by writing a follow-up note to your supervisor after you meet to discuss plans for your leave. Frame it like a thank-you note, although it's more than a courtesy. It's a way of getting your plans in writing so that everyone will be on the same page. Example: "Thank you for meeting with me last week to discuss my maternity leave. As we agreed, I plan to do x, y, and z."

Don't leave it at that. Take the initiative in making sure that everything gets done and everyone concerned understands the plan. Put specific responsibilities, details, and related contact information in writing. Draw up a calendar, if that's useful to your line of work. During your last trimester, meet with your colleagues, assistants, replacements, supervisors, and anyone else who needs to be in the loop about your plans.

Be courteous to the poor souls left behind by keeping an especially tidy desk, well-organized files, and the like from mid-pregnancy on. Even if neatness is not your true nature, doing so will make things easier on everyone. You don't know which day you'll go into labor or whether an unplanned emergency will require you to leave work earlier than expected.

Should I offer to stay in touch or be otherwise available to colleagues during my leave (or when I'm on bed rest)?
It may seem politically savvy—or just the nice thing to do—but staying in close contact with your workplace when you're supposed to be home is usually bad business for you and your

baby. A medical or maternity leave is your right, and for good reasons. These weeks are a tiny portion of your life, and they're supposed to be dedicated to your well being and your baby's.

Advance planning can reduce much of the need to remain in touch. Make your preferences about being contacted clear before you leave. If you don't want to seem uncooperative, you could say, "If there's a dire emergency, of course you know where to reach me. But I'd prefer to spend those few weeks alone with my baby. Here's the plan that should answer all the questions that might come up." Work out, with your colleagues and your supervisor, exactly how your workload will be redistributed. Write memos and have group meetings about the plan, so that no one's left in the dark.

If the faxes, phone calls, and FedEx deliveries persist after you're home, handle them gently yet firmly. Let your answering service or machine pick up telephone messages instead of answering yourself. (If someone asks why you ignore your phone, you can say that you've turned down the ringer so you don't disturb the baby's rest.) Resist the impulse to check your e-mail on the hour or to respond immediately to a fax or package. Dragging your heels a bit reinforces the idea that work is not your number-one priority right now. It may be that your workmates are nervous about your absence. After a few days, they'll begin to realize that the world will go ahead without you for a while.

If you just can't help yourself about continuing to work, nobody's going to stop you—but remember most women don't have a baby more than a handful of times in their lives. Enjoy it!

Exception: If you are home on bed rest and going stir-crazy, and your doctor gives you his blessing to work a little, none of the above applies. In that situation, work may be a pleasant respite from boredom and worry.

What if I change my mind about maternity leave in midstream—say, I want longer leave, or don't want to come back at all?
It's impossible to predict how you'll feel about juggling work and baby until you're in that spot. Thinking about it while you're pregnant is not the same as thinking about it while your baby is in your arms day after day. Some women are sure that they will return to work, only to resign suddenly as the end of their leave draws near. Others plan to stay home, but quickly grow bored or feel a financial strain and find either full- or part-time work. Still others search for a middle ground, perhaps working three days a week or on a graduated schedule of increasing hours as the baby grows older.

Any of these choices is legitimate. To be most fair to your employer and to make it easier on pregnant women who come after you, it's best to be up front if you're not absolutely sure whether you want to return to full-time work or not. Acting absolutely certain, if you're not, would be a misguided show of loyalty. Better to be frank with your supervisor: "I am planning to return, but I may also want to explore part-time options for a few months."

SMALL TALK

How much can I talk about my pregnancy at work?
Less is more when it comes to pregnancy talk in the workplace. It's obvious enough to everyone who sees you that you're having a baby. There's little benefit in regaling your coworkers with tales of your swollen ankles, your sudden absentmindedness, or your debates with your mate over what to name the baby. Save those conversations for lunch breaks and best friends.

Ditto for rubbing your belly in meetings, taking your shoes off to ease discomfort, and lying down on your office floor to catnap.

Remember that you set the tone. If you place your professional image before your pregnant one, others are more likely to follow suit. This can be hard for some women, because, after all, it's fun to obsess about pregnancy when you're expecting. But too much baby talk wastes time. It will ultimately rub your reputation the wrong way. It's not that you have to deny your pregnancy completely; it's a question of scale.

What if everyone else wants to talk *only* about my pregnancy?

A certain amount of pregnancy-related conversation is inevitable. Some co-workers can't help themselves. In fact, they think they're being polite, rather than rude, by constantly querying, "How are you feeling today?" "Are you sure you're comfortable in that chair?" "Hey, you shouldn't be eating those french fries, you know."

Your best response is to not take the bait. Simply say, "I'm fine" and steer the conversation to a business-related discussion. Be persistent yourself.

What's the appropriate reply when a colleague says something really embarrassing?

Some men, especially, can't resist making unfortunate comments to their pregnant colleagues. Perhaps it's because they're embarrassed themselves—although one can't imagine why, since pregnant women are hardly rare birds in workplaces these days. Let the comment pass, if you can, particularly if it seems to have been thoughtlessly uttered. ("You sure are eating for two." "That's a big dress you have there.") Or let it go with a raised eyebrow, a slight frown, or a "Pardon me?" Drawing more attention to his comment will only compound the awkwardness.

(For more replies to rude comments, see Chapter 2, "Busybodies.")

Some of the talk can be downright tactless. One woman was aghast to hear a subordinate exclaim, "Wow! You're getting as big as a horse!" Speechless, she posted the following note on her door:

Things not to say to a pregnant lady:
"Wow, you're getting as big as a horse."
"You look like you are about to pop."
"Make way for the fat lady."

What is more appropriate? Any of the following:
"How are you?"
"Lovely weather we are having."
"Isn't it a beautiful day?"
"Hi."

When They Say...	*You Can Say...*
"Let me carry that briefcase for you."	"I'm not disabled, I'm pregnant."
"And how is Mommy today?"	"I am not your mommy."

What They Say . . .	*You Can Say . . .*
"Can I bring you a few dozen candy bars from the snack bar?"	"No, but you may bring me one, thank you."
"You're not going to get sick in front of the client, are you?"	"Only if your presentation isn't as bad as it was the last time."
"Gee, how can you concentrate on your work?"	"Not very well when you keep interrupting me."
"What if you go into labor right here?"	"Then you'd be the first to know."

ABSENCES

How do I handle frequent disappearances for doctor's appointments?
Frequent checkups are a reality of pregnancy. Your goal should be to minimize lost work time and avoid drawing even more attention to your pregnant self. Try to arrange early-morning appointments; your doctor's schedule is least likely to be thrown off kilter then. Or make them during lunch. If your lunch hour is flexible, take it early or later, around your appointments. Some doctors' offices allow you to book a series of appointments in advance, enabling you to grab the most convenient times before they are filled.
Be sure that your supervisor is aware of your absences (un-

less they coincide with your entitled breaks) and that your work is covered. Don't make a big, disruptive deal out of your disappearances, and others won't view them resentfully.

Can I turn down travel assignments because I'm pregnant?
The amount and nature of business travel varies. If you're a national salesperson, for example, it may be impractical to halt all travel if you are healthy. Always consult your doctor first. International travel is often frowned on during the first trimester, for example, because the risk of miscarriage is high in early pregnancy. Most airlines refuse to board pregnant passengers in their ninth month. Or there may be other cir-cumstances guiding your specific situation. You will then need to meet with your supervisor to jointly determine what accommodations can be made.

I was once asked to make a stressful overseas trip midway through a pregnancy. Although it was a "safe" time to travel, I didn't feel comfortable about it. Because a previous preg-nancy had ended in miscarriage, my physician offered to write a note recommending against the trip. Ultimately I made a case to my supervisor that I preferred to stay home and offered to take on another assignment in its place. You won't know what's possible until you talk over the pros and cons with others.

EATING

Is it rude to snack in front of coworkers?
Whether to ward off morning sickness or satisfy the near-constant hunger that plagues some women, it's smart to stash nutritious snacks in your desk or the bag you carry to work. Now that "desk-fasting" (eating breakfast at your desk) is in vogue for the hyperscheduled worker, no one may look

askance. If it's the sort of workplace where no one nibbles openly all day, however, do so on the sly. Avoid noshing during meetings (one on one or in a group).

The best snack choices are easy to eat surreptitiously, require little preparation, don't smell up the office, and don't make disruptive noise (as do potato chips, which aren't the best for you anyway). Good choices: dry cereal, raisins, sunflower seeds, snack-sized crackers, trail mix, granola bars, bananas, sliced apples, crudités (such as raw carrot or celery sticks), bottled water; juice boxes. Keep the snacks out of sight. Juice bottles and wrappers littering your desk send a slovenly message, whether you're pregnant or not.

Is it cool to send an intern or a messenger out to get a fix for my cravings?

If it would be normal to send an underling to fetch food if you weren't pregnant, there's no reason why you can't do the same now. (You don't have to explain the "why" behind the errand.) But if having assistants run such errands is not one of your usual job perks, you're better off buying the pickles and Fritos yourself.

Is it rude for colleagues to order wine at lunch in the presence of a pregnant coworker?

Just because one person can't have alcohol (or coffee, or sushi, or steak tartare), it doesn't follow that the whole office must abstain. It would not, for example, be considered rude to order dessert in the presence of a diabetic. The pregnant woman knows what she's supposed to eat or not eat, and presumably her baby's health is strong enough motivation for her to dine around her temporary restrictions for a few months.

Exception: If a colleague has recently quit smoking because she's pregnant, and is finding this to be difficult, it's considerate not to light up in front of her. More than merely trying to avoid a favored substance, she's trying to break an addiction. She can use all the help she can get.

WORK SHOWERS

Should colleagues throw a shower for an expectant mother?
Though the expectant mom shouldn't expect one, an office shower is a nice gesture. It could be women-only or coed, depending on your workplace dynamics. Limit the guests to immediate colleagues (as opposed to the entire workplace); the last thing you want to have are grumbly well-wishers who feel obligated, due to office politics, to attend yet another shower where they barely know the honoree. To avoid offending anyone, circulate a memo to those in the honoree's department; guests can attend as they choose.

A lunch at a restaurant is easiest and least disruptive. Guests pay for their own meals and pool resources to treat the mom-to-be. The conference room is a great locale for a surprise shower because it provides a ready-made pretext for getting the honoree there. At a work shower it's appropriate, if desired, to buy a group gift, an option more convenient and perhaps less expensive for guests than individual gifts.

If your workplace frowns on such social displays (or is a family-unfriendly dinosaur that would rather not be reminded of one of its workers' impending maternity leave), close colleagues could band together to have a small off-site luncheon as a shower, or arrange to meet mom and baby for lunch after she delivers. Showers for dads-to-be are a new twist. The same general rules apply.

Should one's boss be invited to the baby shower?
Depending on the mom-to-be's relationship with her immediate supervisor, it may be appropriate to extend an

invitation—but it's not necessary or even expected. Nor is a boss obligated to attend an employee's shower, if he or she is invited, because it is a personal event.

Exception: If it's an office shower held by coworkers at the workplace, it's good politics to include the supervisor in the festivities.

HOW LONG TO WORK

Is it gauche to work up until the last minute?
There's nothing wrong with working until you go into labor. In fact, many moms prefer it to sitting around the house waiting for labor to begin. If you arbitrarily select a last-day date two weeks before your due date, say, and then your baby is two weeks late, that's one month without a job or a baby. If you're planning to return to work, you'd probably rather have that month of leave time for baby-tending.

LABOR AT WORK

I'm afraid I'll go into labor at the office—should I be expected to be graceful under that kind of pressure?
For ninety-nine out of a hundred women, labor does not start à la Lucy Ricardo or Didi (*Rugrats*) Pickles, where you suddenly clutch your midsection and howl, "Omigod, it's time!" The most dramatic thing that might happen is that your water will break, and this is the exception, not the norm. (Nor are severe contractions likely to immediately begin even if your water does break.)

For most first-time moms, labor starts as a gradually felt series of contractions that grow ever more intense. Especially with first-time mothers, the intensity builds fairly slowly.

That should give you plenty of warning to pack up and go home.

If you're really concerned, develop an emergency plan. Have your partner carry a pager or cell phone so he can be in constant touch. Or designate a close colleague to be the person who'll help you home or to your doctor's. Again, be discreet—you don't need to whip the whole office into a frenzy. Nor do you probably want all eyes on you, nine months huge and panicky to boot.

THE BIG NEWS

How should the office find out about the birth?
You or your partner should call your supervisor (or his or her assistant) when making the initial flurry of calls from the hospital. That's preferable to just letting one of your office buddies know and asking her to pass along word to your boss for you.

Should colleagues send a baby gift after the child is born?
Word of a baby's birth ought to be greeted with a personal note of congratulations from the supervisor, at minimum. Co-workers don't have to send individual wishes, unless they're good friends. A boss is not obligated to send more than a note when an employee has a new baby. Some employers do send flowers, gift baskets, or a collective gift. All are thoughtful gestures that the grateful parents are likely to long remember.

Do's and Don'ts For Colleagues

DO ask when she's due or how long she plans to work, once you've issued hearty congratulations.

DO NOT *say, "Gee, I never thought of you as the maternal type," or "I hope you're not expecting me to cover for you while you're gone."*

DO proceed with business as usual; your pregnant co-worker is not going to drop the baby right in front of you.

DO NOT *ask any personal or nosy questions, including how much weight she's gained; whether she plans to have natural childbirth, or her views on circumcision.*

DO look her in the eyes, not the midsection, when talking to her.

DO NOT *place your hand on her belly during a really boring meeting so that you can feel the baby move.*

DO promote her if you had already been planning to do so.

DO NOT *try to predict what you think her workload or her efficiency will be like after the baby arrives; that's her business.*

DO offer her the most comfortable chair first, if there's a choice of seating.

DO NOT *dramatically flatten yourself against a wall when she walks past in the hallway; nobody's that big.*

DO let her carry on her usual workload—if she needs do anything differently in light of her condition, she'll let you know.
DO NOT *keep her away from visiting clients or VIPs; rest assured they've all seen pregnant women before.*

DO feel free to tell her that her new dress or haircut look great, without reference to her pregnant state.
DO NOT *ask why her blazer doesn't button.*

DO your share graciously if you are on the team helping to ensure the transition of work responsibilities during her maternity leave.
DO NOT *privately bellyache that family-friendly work policies discriminate against childless people. It's attitudes like that that have made the United States one of the least child-friendly countries in the developed world—which is ultimately a bad thing for us all.*

DO send a congratulatory note after the baby's born (especially if you're the boss).
DO NOT *add a postscript that says, "Miss you already; please hurry back!"*

DO let her know that she's missed while she's on maternity leave but that "everything's under control."
DO NOT *enviously confuse her maternity leave with vacation, unless you consider sleep deprivation, leaky breasts, sitz baths, and two hours preparation just to get to the grocery store to be your idea of vacation.*

DO make sure there's a comfortable, private place in the office where she can pump breast milk upon her return, if necessary.

DO NOT *borrow milk from the office fridge for your morning coffee before carefully reading the label.*

6

Baby Showers

Mothers-to-be often face the prospect of baby showers with a mixture of excitement and dread. Excitement, because this special party is one of the big rituals of new motherhood. It's fun—not to mention easy—to sit back and be the guest of honor. It's nice to be supported by your loved ones at such an emotional time. And all those baby clothes and blankets are still more tangible proof that your baby's almost here!

But apprehension is common, too. There you are, in your superripe state, being asked to be a ready target for all that clucking and belly-patting and advice-doling. If you're someone who has had little experience with babies, you may feel all the more sheepish about all the fuss (not to mention embarrassed that you can't identify half the alien gifts—lap pads? wipes warmers?). It won't help matters if your memories of showers you've attended in the past were either long, dull affairs or cornfests full of excruciatingly silly games.

The good news about a baby shower is that no two are just alike. As a tradition, they're relatively young, a twentieth-century invention. So there are no hard-and-fast rules. Also, the honoree usually gets a fair say in what sort of celebration she'd most prefer. Most of all, they're an occasion to celebrate your baby-to-be. So when someone offers to host your baby shower, thank them graciously and enjoy yourself.

HOSTING A SHOWER

Who may host a baby shower?

Ideally, anyone except an immediate relative of the mom-to-be. Why not a close relation? Because it looks like you're sending your family out clamoring for gifts on your behalf. That rules out the mom-to-be's mother or sister. Mothers-in-law and sisters-in-law fall into the gray zone; traditional etiquette says they should not be hostesses either. More distant relations—aunts, cousins—are fine.

But there are always exceptions. In some families, sisters (including sisters-in-law and stepsisters) organize showers without anyone thinking ill of them. Showers are commonly hosted jointly—a friend may team up with a relative, for example. Especially if the party is large, cohosting shares the expenses and the work, which can be considerable.

If family members throwing a baby shower is traditional in your circle, and no guest would find it odd, that's one thing. But if in doubt, let friends take the lead.

I hate to put my family or friends to any trouble—can I host my own baby shower?

Never. Even folks who wouldn't think anything amiss if your mother held the shower would find the idea of a self-thrown shower too greedy and self-involved. But don't worry—someone's bound to step forward to offer to do the job. What you can do, very properly, is to air your preferences about the event. Your host(s) should solicit your opinion about when to have it and whom to invite. Also give your thoughts about what kind of shower you'd like—a big family-and-friends bash with quirky games; a cozy, gossipy lunch with girlfriends;

an elegant couples brunch; whatever. You deserve a party. Moreover, you deserve to have it suit your tastes.

GUESTS

Who should be invited?
Only good friends and family members should be on the guest list, since shower-goers are expected to bring a gift. The hostess should draw up the guest list in concert with the honoree.

Grandmothers-to-be should refrain from urging invitations to every one of their friends for whose children they've bought gifts over the years, unless those friends also know the mother-to-be.

Should out-of-town friends and relatives be invited, so they don't feel left out?
It's not necessary to invite distant friends and relatives to a baby shower unless you are sure a person will be in town. Because of the distance, they probably don't expect an invitation. Nor should faraway friends feel "left out" by not receiving one. If the honoree or her hostess suspect that someone might expect an invite because they are very close to the parents-to-be, though, it's perfectly fine to call her and ask whether she plans to make a special trip. Some people find it fun to surprise an honoree with their unexpected presence at a baby shower. You just have to play it by ear.

Anyone who receives an invitation to a shower that she can't attend is not, however, obligated to send a gift in her absence. Since the purpose of a shower is to assemble baby items for the parents, that's reason enough not to invite those who are unlikely to come because they live far away.

Are men supposed to be invited, in these enlightened times? If you want to have them—and if they want to come—the dad-to-be and his male buddies are certainly welcome at baby showers today. Those are two big "ifs" however. It's true that most modern dads jump in and attend childbirth classes, cut the umbilical cord, and change diapers—but few guys like to sit around listening to old wives' tales while unwrapping onesies.

A shower, after all, is a girl thing. It's a time for women to gather together and exchange labor stories and coo over stuffed bunnies and teeny tiny clothing. A baby shower is the initiation meeting for the Motherhood Club. Many women don't *want* their mates in tow, turning pale during the labor stories and making wisecracks when the Diaper Genie is unwrapped. Therefore no dad-to-be should take offense if he is excluded from the proceedings. This may be the dawn of the twenty-first century, but showers are one of the ultimate traditions—nice when updated but also acceptable if left as is.

That's one viewpoint, anyway. Another perspective is that the baby is being welcomed into a new family, so why not make a shower a family affair? After all, both parents will raise the child. Assigning rigid male-female roles to new parenthood (she goes to the shower; he passes out the cigars) is considered by some to be a throwback to the days when dads paced outside the delivery room. Thus, dual-sex showers are increasingly common, reflecting dads' active participation in babyrearing.

Many men are flattered to be included. When both parents are invited to the shower, men should also be on the guest list. Coed showers are usually buffet suppers or picnics, rather than afternoon teas or luncheons.

WHEN TO HOLD

When should a baby shower be held?
Traditionally, a baby shower is held during the last weeks of pregnancy. It should be held late enough so that the baby is clearly healthy and growing and the mother is really showing—but not so late that the baby might arrive before the shower guests do. About three to six weeks before the due date is the usual window. (Cut it closer than that at your own risk: My baby shower was scheduled exactly three weeks before my due date—but I wound up calling my hostess to say I couldn't make it from a hospital room. My daughter chose to be born that morning.)

The benefits of having a shower before the baby's arrival are numerous. First-time parents have to acquire all their baby gear. Buying a layette and all the other things a newborn requires is much easier to do during the pregnancy than with a baby in tow. Also, by having the shower first, the items can be used immediately after the birth. A shower can also be a welcome break in the monotony of waiting that sets in for expectant moms around the seventh or eighth month.

A "welcome baby" shower after the birth is another option. This is preferred by families who follow a superstition against acquiring anything for the baby until he or she is safely born. It's also an option for women who have medical difficulties (such as those requiring bed rest) that make a big hoopla inconvenient. If you have a shower after the birth, you're apt to receive more personalized and gender-specific items. You can also show off your baby to your guests.

The shower's hostess should plan the date in concert with the mom-to-be, working as far in advance as possible and around her schedule. The hostess needs to give herself enough time to arrange the details and mail the invitations (up to three weeks in advance of a big party); guests will need ample time to clear their calendars and to plan and buy their presents.

What time of day works best?
Typically showers are held on:

- weekday evenings (after work hours)
- weekend afternoons (after giving guests a chance to run errands, attend church, and so on)
- during weekday lunch hours (for coworkers or small groups)

About two hours is enough time.

Are surprise parties okay?
Opinions are divided about the wisdom of this type of shower. The answer may depend on the personality of the honoree.

The rationale against surprises: Some women don't welcome being thrown for a loop—waking up every day with a changing body is surprising enough. Especially in late pregnancy, a woman may not be feeling her best, or think that she looks her best without giving extra care to her makeup or dress. To be thrust into the spotlight without having a chance to prepare isn't fair. If it's a surprise, the party planners can't get her input on the guest list, which can be useful if she's having multiple showers and doesn't want the same people to feel they need to give gifts more than once. Also, when the shower is kept secret from the mom-to-be, she may begin to feel forgotten or ignored, which puts her in an uncomfortable and awkward position, since she can't very well go around asking, "Hey guys, what about my shower?"

The rationale favoring a surprise: Originally, baby showers

were almost always surprise parties. That removed all element of the honoree feeling that she was "asking" for gifts. Many women love a surprise. For them, an unexpected party—especially one featuring unexpected out-of-town guests—can be a wonderful late-pregnancy pick-me-up. You can get around the frumpy-grumpy honoree dilemma by getting her to the shower via some ruse that requires her to get dressed up, such as a restaurant lunch or a shopping outing.

A surprise shower would also be appropriate at work, say as a small restaurant lunch or meeting-room get-together before her leave begins.

One neat surprise-shower idea that causes no inconvenience to the honoree is the shower-by-mail. When a mom-to-be lives far from her family and friends, they can band together to send her packages during a predetermined time period. Or the gifts can all be sent via overnight mail to arrive on one day.

INVITATIONS

What kind of invitations should be used?
Telephone invitations are fine for very small gatherings. But if there are more than half a dozen invitees, it's best to commit the details to paper. Essential details to include:

- Guest of honor's name
- Date of event
- Location of event (including address, even if you suspect people are familiar with it)
- Starting and ending times
- Guest response information (either RSVP or "Regrets only")
- The host's name and telephone number

Optional information includes:

- The honoree's due date
- The baby-to-be's gender (if known)
- The type of shower (if there is a theme)

The hostess should remember to give an invitation to the guest of honor, to save in her child's baby book, if she wishes.

Commercial fill-in-the-blank invitations are widely available and are by far the quickest way to go. Even less expensive are those the hostess makes on her home computer. Invitations also may be printed up in a print shop. Or if the host is the creative type, scissors and glue can work wonders. Look for good-quality colored paper at office-supply stores, art-supply shops, or stationers.

Consider personalizing the invitation. When I was working as a magazine editor, a friend worded her invitations as "a baby shower honoring Paula Spencer and Baby TK," (TK being journalistic slang for part of the story still "to come").

For a photo buff's baby shower, the invitations featured a silhouette of the honoree with a camera, surrounded by pictures of babies cut out of magazines. Inside it said, "Since Liz is developing a baby, I am developing a baby shower for her . . ."

More variations:

- *She's ready to pop.* Cut out individual small bubbles from bubble wrap and glue one onto the center of a piece of paper. This is the honoree's bulging belly. Draw the rest of her around it.
- *Raining babies.* Draw a picture of an umbrella, or cut out the shape of one from fabric or colored paper. Glue it to the front of the invitation, then, using a rubber stamper of a baby, stamp lots of babies falling down from the sky around the umbrella.

- *Famous babies.* If you live near a museum (or a mall with a museum shop) look for art postcards featuring babies or mothers and babies. Write the invitation information on the back, and forgo envelopes and added postage.
- *Warm fuzzies.* Make teddy bears out of bits of fuzzy fabric, available at fabric stores. Perfect for a teddy-bear shower.
- *First footprints.* Cut out the shape of a baby's foot and write the party information on it. Handprints work, too.
- *Paper dolls.* Look in children's bookstores, toy stores, or novelty shops for infant paper dolls you can use as invitations. Or cut out your own old-fashioned chain of paper dolls (perfect when multiples are due).
- *Diaper time.* Cut and fold a piece of white paper to resemble a diaper, which opens up to reveal the facts. Or use white handkerchiefs to achieve the same result, with the actual invitation wrapped inside.
- *A very personalized invite.* Snap a (flattering) photo of the honoree great with child and use a scanned version of it to illustrate a computer-generated invite. Or obtain photos of the expectant parents when *they* were babies to use in the same way.

LOCATION

Where should a baby shower take place?
Because there is no proscribed format for a shower, there's no single proper setting. Choices include the same as for any party: a private home, a restaurant, a supper club, a reception hall, a public park, and so on. It's best if the locale isn't the expectant mother's home, since she is not the hostess, unless she's on bed rest and can't leave her home.

HOW MANY?

How many showers can I have?

Most women have just one, but more are possible if the mom-to-be has different circles of friends. Her relatives may want to be part of one shower, for example, her coworkers another, her church friends or book club yet another.

The only restriction regarding the number of baby showers a mother may have: The same people should not be invited repeatedly. If this seems unavoidable (for instance, you have a coworker who's also in your Sunday school class and both groups are throwing showers), you could tactfully suggest that the two parties collaborate on one event. If this is not possible or if there are just a few individuals who will be invited twice, single out those people and personally urge them not to bring gifts both times. The friends can then decide whether they want to bring a gift to just one shower (which is perfectly acceptable), or bring a gift to one and a small token to another, or give twice. No one should be expected to give more than once.

Note to party planners: To avoid duplicate invitees, it's wise to consult the honoree when making up the guest list and to invite only those people whom she suggests.

WHO HAS A SHOWER?

Can a second-time mother have a shower?

Because the purpose of a shower is to help new parents accumulate all the bibs and booties they'll need for parenthood but aren't likely to already own, this party was invented for first-time parents. Baby showers first flourished in the postwar baby boom. Babies—and baby gear—were suddenly plentiful. Also, new parents began to live farther from their hometowns than ever and therefore needed help in setting up their nurseries. Borrowed from the already well-established wedding showers, the idea of feting new parents (and for manufacturers, encouraging consumption) was an easy leap.

Presumably by the second go-round, there's not much left that your friends and relatives need to furnish you with. A replay of the first big fest at each subsequent birth begins to feel superfluous. Friends who are likely to send a baby gift to welcome Little Deux are liable to feel resentful if they are expected to buy shower presents as well.

But exceptions abound. If a woman's children are very widely spaced, say seven or more years apart, many of her baby things may have been given away or are out of date, leaving her in need of replacements. Also if a mother has moved to a new area and has many new friends, a second-baby shower can be a lovely welcoming event—and a chance for her to socialize with other moms.

Ultimately, showers are not just about giving goods; they're also about celebrating pregnancy. Smaller celebrations among close friends to acknowledge the impending birth are both sweet and thoughtful. Think festive lunch or tea party with a small number of guests and few, if any, pull-out-all-the-stops party games. Gifts are not necessary; camaraderie is.

Can a single mother have a shower?

Unwed mothers are in as much in need of baby items as married mothers are. A baby shower has nothing to do with one's marital status. If you're concerned about being a target for whispers or lectures about the absence of the baby's father, don't invite anyone who would be unable to maintain the proper spirit at the shower.

If the mom-to-be previously had a big shower for a baby she lost, should she have another shower for her second pregnancy?
Yes, if the previous gifts were returned. The mother still needs items for her new baby. Often a mother who has had a late miscarriage or a stillbirth prefers that a subsequent child's baby shower be held after the delivery, even though the risk of a repeat of her tragedy is minute. Even if the gifts weren't returned, a small party is nice.

Should a shower be thrown for a woman who's following the tradition of not buying anything for the baby until it is born?
Yes, the superstitious mother deserves a shower as much as the next mom—but to respect her wishes, the celebration should be scheduled for after her delivery. This is a tradition with its roots in the days when pregnancy outcomes were iffier than they are today. Parents chose not to make too much fuss over the baby until its health and well-being were assured. Some parents still hate to "jinx" the pregnancy by celebrating too early.

Can a shower be thrown only for the father?
This would be a very cutting-edge shower thrown by pretty progressive pals. Which is not to say it couldn't be done, or couldn't be a great time. Sometimes officemates (men and women) throw such a party for their colleague.

Do I have to have a shower at all?
No. A shower is meant to be happy and fun (both for you and those who attend it). An offer to host one for you is a warm act of friendship for which a pregnant woman ought to feel grateful. It's also an efficient (and no-cost) way to outfit your nursery. But no one's going to force you to have one. If you

want to be a spoilsport, that's your prerogative. Do deliver warm thanks to the person who offers to throw one when you decline.

WORK SHOWERS

Aren't showers held at work unprofessional?
In general, a mom-to-be shouldn't fear that a bit of celebrating about her new baby will make her look less competent in her employer's eyes. The shower's tone should match the general way your office celebrates other commemorative milestones, such as birthdays or retirements. For example, if celebrations tend to take place "off campus" at a restaurant during lunch, or in the meeting room at the end of the day, it would be appropriate for the shower to follow suit.

(For more on working-mom-to-be showers, see Chapter 5, "At Work.")

GRANDMOTHER SHOWERS

Are grandmother showers in good taste?
Who wouldn't love a party where all the guests bring presents? Showers were once limited to brides and expectant mothers, but lately they're held for all sorts of passages: young adults furnishing their first apartments, unmarried couples moving into a new house, and yes, women about to become grandmothers. The latter idea sprang up as a way for a grandmother-to-be's friends to fete her and give a present (or presents) to her expected grandchild. A grandmother shower is most often given when the woman and her friends live far away from the mother-to-be or when the friends don't know the mom-to-be very well.

The get-together should be intimate, among close friends

only. The gifts should be for the baby or for the grandmother-to-be to use while caring for the baby (such as an extra umbrella stroller or books). It should not be a droll, mean-spirited now-you're-over-the-hill sort of party. Nor should it bear any traditional shower trappings (games, favors, and the like). Such festivities are reserved for the woman who's actually having the baby—who, by the way, is not usually on the guest list at a grandmother's shower. (Otherwise it would be a shower for *her*.)

THEMES

Does a baby shower need a theme?
Unlike birthday parties or balls, baby showers come with a built-in theme: babies. But that obvious fact needn't limit a host from embellishing it. Ambitious hosts can create a memorable event by inventing a unifying theme for the invitations, the decorations, and possibly even the refreshments and entertainment.
Some ideas:

- *All pink and blue.* Use these two colors (or one of them, if the baby's gender is known) for balloons, plates, streamers, and even refreshments. Set pink plates on a blue tablecloth, or vice versa. Tie pastel balloons to chair backs. Serve pink lemonade, pinkish tomato bisque, and blueberry cobbler or baby-blue-tinted cookies or cakes. For place cards, fill clear four-ounce baby bottles with pink and blue jelly beans and write guests' names on clear tape attached to the bottles. (The tape can be removed later and the bottles given to the new mom.)
- *Teddy-bear brigade.* Find invitations that picture a bear. Invite guests to bring their own childhood bears. Make

a teddy centerpiece out of them (put the bears in diapers to reinforce the baby-shower theme). Use a beautifully illustrated copy of Goldilocks and the Three Bears as the guest register for guests to sign; present it to the honoree as Baby's first book. Ideal for teddy lovers. Fun twist: Give the mom-to-be a lacy teddy of her own (the lingerie kind) to wear post-baby and remind her that she'll have her old body back again eventually.

- *Baby dolls.* As with the teddy bear shower, invite guests to bring their childhood baby dolls. Set them up in wicker prams and rocking chairs in a corner of the room. At discount stores or party stores, you can find tiny, inexpensive baby dolls to use as table favors or to attach to napkin rings. Carry the theme to invitations and place cards by using pictures of babies cut out from parenting magazines.

- *Raining babies.* Use raingear as the decorative theme. Umbrella motifs are usually easy to find on baby-shower invitations, paper plates and napkins, and wrapping papers. Prop the real thing against walls or hang a few from the ceiling. Make a centerpiece out of shiny rain hats onto which are taped pictures of babies. Add tiny paper parasols (available at party stores and liquor stores) to drinks. Make the first gift opened by the mom-to-be an umbrella stroller.

- *Welcome to the nursery.* This is a fresh and easy way to decorate. Scatter childhood icons (borrowed from a guest with children or brand-new, as a gift to the honoree) on the tables: Duplo blocks, stuffed animals, rattles, dolls, and the like. Or add baby items, such as bottles, diaper pins, and pacifiers. Use wooden blocks to spell out guests' names as placecards. Baby blankets or quilts, covered with a clear plastic sheet if necessary, can serve as tablecloths. Use large bibs as place mats. Display the gifts in a pram or cradle. Play lullabies as background music.

- *Ready to hatch.* Think fertility, chicks and eggs. Send egg-shaped invites: "Please come to a party for Marge before she hatches." Make it a brunch and serve egg-based dishes. Dye pink and blue hard-boiled eggs Easter-style for a centerpiece. Play games like spoon races—who can carry an egg in a spoon the fastest across a room without dropping or breaking it.
- *Fairy godmothers.* Take a page from *Sleeping Beauty.* Send invitations that look like advertisements for "fairy godmothers" for the baby, and include a pinch of fairy dust (glitter) to spill from the envelope when it's opened. Decorate with a fairy motif (angels make suitable winged stand-ins). Sprinkle glitter on the table. Make or buy magic wands adorned with each guest's name as place markers. Pass around a beautifully decorated blank book in which each guest godmother writes down the skill or trait that she intends to teach the newborn as he or she grows—redeemable in the future. And hope that Maleficent doesn't show up.
- *Garden party.* Most pregnant women bloom. Since the mother is being celebrated as much as the baby, many women appreciate a luncheon that's simply beautiful. Use floral-patterned dishes (or floral paper ware) and floral tablecloths and napkins. Adorn the table with a fresh centerpiece, and place bud vases at each setting. Hothouse spring flowers for a fall or winter shower are especially beautiful and have a fresh "new" scent. You could even ask all the guests to wear floral dresses or blouses.
- *High tea.* Skip all the gimmicks, if it's more to the taste of the hostess and the honoree. Instead, prepare a lovely, lavish tea party—complete with lacy white linens (no paper napkins). Polish the best silver and get out that wedding-gift china and crystal. Brew good loose tea and

serve it out of pretty teapots with traditional tea fare: cucumber sandwiches, tea biscuits, scones and clotted cream, and fresh strawberries.

Clever Corsages

Designate the Mom of Honor with a corsage made from one of the following:

- A pacifier hung from pink and blue ribbons
- A pair of newborn-sized booties or socks
- A soft fabric rattle attached with a diaper pin
- Her name (or "Mom") strung from small letter blocks (available at many toy shops). Or make a necklace from the same
- A pink or blue name tag that reads "Mom-to-Be," pinned on with a pastel diaper pin. (This idea can be adapted for all guests' name tags at large showers where everyone may not be acquainted.)

GIFTS

What are appropriate shower gifts?
The object of a shower is to help the mother assemble all the dozens of little things she'll need for a small person who isn't even here yet. Therefore old-school etiquette holds that the gifts should be tokens (bibs, rattles, layette items), with the big presents held off until after the birth. It makes sense that the grander, more personalized, or more lasting objects are given to commemorate the baby's arrival, since it's the more momentous occasion.

Yet strollers and automatic baby swings have become shower-gift standards today. Even if this is true in your circle of shower-goers, no guest should feel obligated to give something comparatively lavish. Larger gifts are still typically given by close family members or by groups of individuals who have pitched together.

(For a detailed list of shower-gift suggestions, see Chapter 14, "Great Gifts.")

Can a host dictate what sort of gift guests should buy?

Gifts are supposed to be given freely, from the heart—even at showers, where everyone knows the ultimate purpose is to bring a present. You can't demand guests bring a particular item to a baby shower. Not only do guests have individual tastes, but budgets differ, too.

It is possible, however, to plan a shower that has a theme that can naturally extend to the gift giving. Adding this fresh twist is a nice idea when the shower is for a second or third baby, or if you know the mom-to-be is having more than one shower.

The hostess indicates the shower's theme on the invitations: "It's a Peter Rabbit shower, which is what Joan has chosen to furnish the nursery." (Use Peter Rabbit invitations to reinforce the message.) Or, "Please come to a layette shower to help fill Baby's wardrobe." It's up to the guests to take the hint and comply as they wish. They're not obligated to.

Some of the following theme-gift ideas can also be incorporated into traditional showers:

- *Best-advice shower.* Each guest furnishes her personal child-drearing tips, which can be written out and bound into a special book before the shower. (Enclose a three-by-five index card with the invitation.) Spark ideas by encouraging guests to think along the lines of these prompts: "Things I wish someone had told me sooner," "Don't pay any attention when people tell you . . ." or "My best time-saving tactic." This idea works well when there are several generations on the guest list. These "recipes for motherhood" can be presented to the honoree in a recipe card file or bound together in a booklet. For additional gifts, each guest brings the item she found most useful as a new mother. Invite guests to consider items the mom-to-be may not have thought of: Dr. Spock's baby-care guide; a gizmo such as a monitor; nursing clothes for convenient breastfeeding; button-front baby shirts instead of the type that go over a flopsy newborn's head, etc.

- *Baby's first library shower.* Each guest buys a favorite children's book. Choices can include cloth or board "first books," classics such as *Curious George* and Dr. Seuss, Christmas classics, or even books targeted to older children that the baby will grow up to enjoy, such as *The Velveteen Rabbit* or *Charlotte's Web.* This is a great idea for a shower given by a book club or for a teacher. But any expectant parents will appreciate it.

- *Outfit-the-nursery shower.* This is handy for parents on a tight budget. Guests furnish all the details for the baby's room: lamp, crib bumpers, diaper stacker, night-light, mobile, and so on. It's best if the parents have already chosen a nursery theme or color scheme, so that the presents coordinate. This should be noted on the invitation: "It's a (Paddington Bear/Mother Goose/rainbow/choo-choo train) shower."

- *Growing-baby shower.* Guests are asked to help furnish the baby's wardrobe, but each guest (or each two or three guests) is asked to bring a specific size: newborn, three months, six months, nine months, twelve months. This prevents the new mom from having too many adorable clothes during the first weeks, and none at all by the half-year mark. Guests will have to think ahead about the seasons, and of course no one knows whether the baby will be larger or smaller than average. It's therefore best to buy from a shop where exchanges will be easy on the mother, should they be necessary. The packages can all be placed inside a hamper, which is also wrapped (perhaps as a gift from the hostess).

- *The time-of-day shower.* Transfer this wedding-shower staple to inspire guests to think up gifts for babies. In her invitation, each invitee is assigned a particular time of day, 'round the clock, and asked to bring a gift appropriate for that hour. For example, at 10 A.M. a guest might bring a toy or bath towels; at 3 A.M. a sleeper suit or blanket would be appropriate.

- *IOU shower.* Guests bring written "IOU" coupons for services they wish to provide the parents. Examples: baby-sitting services, grocery shopping, housecleaning services, laundry, lawn mowing, chauffeuring the mother to pediatrician appointments, delivery of home-cooked meals.

- *The baby-quilt shower.* Each invitee provides one quilt square to make a blanket for the baby. Obviously this works best when the majority of participants are handy with a needle and thread. But not all squares need to be traditional appliqued quilt patches. They can also be embroidered or cross-stitched designs, painted fabric, knitted or crocheted, or an especially soft or pretty fragment of fabric. One person should be responsible for stitching the pieces together into the whole. Depending on the materials used, the result will either be a baby-safe blanket or a wall decoration for the nursery that can be used as the child gets older. This concept is especially thoughtful when would-be guests are scattered across the country or live far from the honoree and cannot be present at a traditional shower.

- *The handiwork shower.* Here's another idea for gifted seamstresses: Each participant makes a different, coordinating component of the baby's nursery: Crib bumpers, crib sheet, receiving blankets, quilt, decorative pillow, diaper stacker, diaper bag, baby outfit, stuffed animal, even curtains. This could also be a welcome joint gift from a group of friends who all sew. Of course, it's a good idea to consult the honoree in advance about her preferences for fabrics, colors, and decor.

- *The hand-me-down shower.* This works best when most of the mom-to-be's friends are already mothers. Everyone brings clothes, furniture, equipment, or toys that they have used. Obviously, items should be in pristine condition—barely used baby clothes, a repainted changing table, and so on. Nonmothers can join the spirit by giving new life to previously used items, such as framing baby-themed old prints or magazine illustrations for the nursery.

- *The chef shower.* The person organizing this "shower" gives friends and family members a piece of Tupperware or other food-storage container. Each person is assigned a day following the baby's birth to bring the parents a main dish and a side dish. The mom-to-be gets to keep the containers, and is spared the task of returning them to their proper owners. (The dishes can also be brought all at once to a party shortly before delivery, if the honoree has an ample freezer.)

Is it okay to enclose a list of things you really need in the invitation?

In a word, no. Even though everyone knows the purpose of

a shower is to flood an expectant mom with gifts, issuing a list of wants to every guest smacks of blatant greed. The hostess should not even cite the place(s) the parents have registered for baby gifts—it's tantamount to sticking a bridal registry list in with the wedding invitation. Presents should come from the heart, not a ready-made shopping list.

What if you really covet a certain windup baby swing that converts to a high chair and a toddler bed? Or you've decorated your nursery in a Disney Babies motif and want a layette to match? Mention it to your mom and your hostess and let them pass the word when they're asked what you might like. You may also furnish your hosts with a written list of your preferences, as a crib sheet they can refer to when they're asked for suggestions. But this list should not be included in the shower invite itself. If you must register at a store—a widespread practice, although still frowned on by traditionalists— let your friends verbally tell others where.

Why is registering for gifts at a store frowned on?
Gift registries do make things easy on everyone. The mother gets exactly which style of crib sheet or breast pump she prefers and the guests do not have to trouble themselves thinking about what she might like. Stores ranging from big chains like Babies R Us to small children's shops offer gift registries. Some places even allow shoppers to make a donation toward a particular item without having to buy the whole thing.

In fact, gift registries have become so commonplace as to seem almost perfectly acceptable. Nonetheless, there's something depressingly sterile and commercial about the practice. The problem is that the new mom is not supposed to really be sure what she'll need for new motherhood, and the guests are supposed to be showering her with enlightenment. What's more, it's the buyer's prerogative to decide which smocked dress or adorable rattle she wishes to purchase. If she's simply going to fill an order, she may just as well hand over the cold cash instead at the shower.

It's best if everyone approach the occasion in the spirit of spontaneous joy it deserves, rather than as an acquisition-athon. (You can always return things you don't like.)

What about giving pink and blue gifts—are they still standard for babies, or too stereotypical?
In the 1970s and 1980s, the tradition of giving pink for girls and blue for boys dipped in popularity, victim to hypersensitivity over sex stereotyping. There may be old-style feminists out there who still wince at the practice, and if you know this is someone's belief it's polite to respect it. Certainly there's a whole rainbow of beautiful baby clothes to choose from. But the vast majority of parents enjoy the tradition of dressing boys in blue and girls in pink, particularly in the early months.

As traditions go, it's not a particularly ancient one. The pink-and-blue fad was concocted by late-nineteenth-century merchants as a way to sell more clothes. Blue had traditionally been a male color because it carried connotations of spirituality, protectiveness, and strength—the color of workmen's clothing, the color connected with the ancient European sky gods, who were male. Blue clothing was thought to offer a child divine protection. Later, pink may have been chosen for girls because it is a daintier version of that fleshy, passionate and "female" tone, red (and the opposite of cool, celestial blue). Zoologist Desmond Morris points out a folk "explanation" for these color assignments is that boys wore blue because male babies were said to be born in blue cabbage patches, whereas girls were born inside pink roses.

Of course, most parents dress their daughters in blues. But not many American mamas, even those who resist gender stereotypes, choose pink for their sons. *Exception:* Many Oriental cultures are blind to these European color connotations.

If you don't know the baby's gender at the shower, "generic" yellows and pale greens abound. For young babies, white is perhaps the most attractive color of all. Contrary to popular opinion, white clothes are no trouble to keep clean at that age—at least not until the little one starts on strained squash and mudpies.

Can I ask for money instead of gifts?
Granted, this is a new century. It's permissible to drop broad hints about what you'd like to receive. You might register your preferences at a store. You might urge your hostess to list the name of that store in the shower invite. You may even be so brazen as to include the very list of desired items in the invitation's envelope. All of these practices—once frowned on—now have their supporters, and you probably know very nice people who have done all of them.

But one thing no pregnant woman or her hosts may do is to ask for cold cash in lieu of gifts. Neither may your hostess, either in person or by the invitation. It's too cold and calculating—and this is supposed to be a time of warm and fuzzy joy. New moms need lots of miscellaneous baby items, and it's the privilege of your friends and relatives to provide them. What if you don't like what they choose? You can always exchange the items. What if you're broke and need a crib or a stroller? Then your hostess can ask (but never insist) some guests if they'd like to contribute to a large item because you really need it. But don't use your baby-to-be to extort money from those who love you.

It is, by the way, acceptable for a guest to give cash, if she likes, which, while not very original, does always fit and is always of an agreeable color.

TWIN GIFTS

If twins are expected, does each guest bring two gifts? And what about higher-order multiples?
Multiple gifts are thoughtful, and can be cute (say, three co-ordinating receiving blankets). They're not necessary, though. Shower gifts are not supposed to be lavish, so cost is not the issue. Practicality should be. A mother of triplets will be doing laundry three times as often. Therefore three T-shirts, instead of one, are a welcome gift. But if you are giving an item that won't be needed in duplicate or triplicate—say, a diaper pail—then there's no need to come with two other gifts in hand as well. No one's counting.

Should gift cards be read aloud as the gifts are opened?
Since the whole point of a shower is to give gifts, the opening of presents is usually the chief entertainment of the party. Therefore, this shouldn't be done "off to one side" or worse, after the party is over. The honoree should let the other guests know who the gift is from, and either hold it up or pass it around so it can be duly admired by all. Whether she reads aloud a personal message written in the card is up to her.

Are invitees who can't make the shower supposed to send a gift?
Those who send regrets to a hostess are not obligated to also send a present. Nor should the guest of honor expect them to. Close friends or family members who must decline an invitation often want to send something anyway of course. The gift should be mailed ahead in care of the hostess, so that it may be opened at the shower. It can also be mailed

or hand-delivered directly to the honoree before or soon after the shower.

GAMES

How do I break it to my hostess that I don't want to play silly games?
Ideally the mom-to-be should be encouraged to set the overall tone. If she absolutely detests the idea of gimmicky games, they should be avoided or kept to a minimum. But the planner, not the honoree, makes the rules.

Some shower-throwers can't resist quirky games, especially if they've become family rituals. If the fun is sprung on you at your party, be a good sport and go along. It's a baby shower, for goodness sake. It can't hurt—and it might be more fun than you think.

So what are the traditional shower pastimes?
For some folks, the presentation and opening of gifts is ample entertainment. Others prefer more merrymaking. The trick is to let the occasion be festive and sociable without feeling overly programmed. The best baby showers also avoid forcing guests to embarrass themselves. You don't have to have any quirky games at your baby shower—the gathering of friends and simple conversation makes for a pleasant enough time. Or the host can organize one or two such activities to break the ice and get the party rolling. Fortunately, there are many games that manage to lend frivolity without being ridiculous.

Here are some of the classics:

- *You've got the cutest little baby face.* Each guest brings a picture of herself as a baby. The host mounts them all on a single large piece of cardboard or poster board, and writes a numeral next to each. Guests are then invited to match each baby with a corresponding grown-up. Whoever gets the most right is the winner.

- *Name that taste.* Guests are given spoons and paper plates onto which have been drawn several small, numbered circles. The host brings out assorted jars of baby foods (the pureed, strained kind), with the labels removed or obscured. She places a small amount of the first type onto the circle on the each guest plate numbered "one," and continues until each circle has been filled with a different kind of baby food. Guests then guess what each type of food is and write down their answers. Whoever gets the best scores wins. (Choose a colorful variety: peas, squash, rice cereal, mixed vegetables, beef, and so on.)

- *Know your baby items.* There are two versions to this game, which features familiar small baby-care objects: teething ring, diaper, rectal thermometer, diaper wipes, pacifier, nail clippers, nasal aspirator, and the like. For the first version, a collection of thirty or more such items are assembled on a large tray. Guests have thirty seconds to memorize everything they see. They then write down all the items that they remember. The best memory wins. For the second version, familiar baby items are placed, one at a time, in a brown paper bag or cloth sack. Guests feel inside the sack and try to identify the mystery object.

- *Brand X.* Each guest is given a folded piece of paper on which the brand name of a popular baby item has been written. Go around the room and ask each person to identify the product. Examples: NUK (nipples); Similac (formula); Luvs (diapers); Balmex (diaper rash ointment); Lansinoh (lanolin for breastfeeding); Graco (strollers, high chairs). This can be a good icebreaker for gatherings featuring older women who may not recognize today's pediatric brands—but are bound to make some hilarious guesses.

- *Baby needs a name.* The honoree picks a letter of the alphabet and a gender. Within an allotted time period (thirty to sixty seconds), guests try to come up with as many baby names as possible. The person who thinks up the most names wins. Variations: Have each guest draw eight children's alphabet blocks or Scrabble game tiles from a basket (without peeking) and, Scrabble-style, come up with a proposed first and middle name for the baby. When everyone has finished, the mom-to-be picks her favorite.

- *How big is Baby?* Start with a large cord of string or ribbon. Pass it and a pair of scissors around, asking each guest to cut the string at a length that would match the circumference of the mom's belly. The winner is the person who estimates the closest match. This game requires a mom-to-be who's a very good sport.

- *Name that nursery rhyme.* Leaf through a book of Mother Goose nursery rhymes to come up with quiz questions you can ask guests. Examples: Who would eat no lean? (Jack Sprat's wife.) Who ran away with the spoon? (The dish.) A light icebreaker.

- *Betcha can't say "baby".* Each guest is given a diaper pin on arrival. Every time someone says "baby," the person who calls it first gets to collect that guest's diaper pin. The object is to collect the most pins by the end of the shower.

Should there be prizes for the winners of shower games?
Most shower games are wacky enough that the fun lies in the playing, not the winning. If used, gifts should be small tokens, such as candy or pink and blue pens. If all the participants are mothers of young children, you could give inexpensive playthings, such as crayons or bathtubs toys. Or you could go

the humor route, awarding home-pregnancy tests, cigars (chocolate or real), and boxes of animal crackers. Another idea: Make all of the prizes of the "baby" theme: Beanie Babies, Baby Ruth candy bars, Sugar Babies candies, Baby Bee brand toiletries, baby wipes, baby-doll nightie, a copy of the movie *Babe*, and the like.

Baby-Shower Table Favors

At a sit-down shower, it's thoughtful to place a small token at each guest's place setting. The favor can tie in with the overall shower theme, or be something that simply extends the festive, lovely mood of the day. You may also incorporate place cards with the favor if you are pre-determining the seating of a large group. Some ideas:

- Small plant or herb in a terra-cotta pot painted to match the table setting
- Flowers in a small ceramic vase or clear glass vase painted with pink and blue trim
- A single stem in a bud vase, or a spray of baby's breath
- Miniature floral arrangement placed in an antique floral teacup (place stems in wet florist's foam)
- Miniature picture frame with the guest's name on a card in place of a photograph
- A votive candle, store-bought or made from a clean (empty) baby-food jar
- Pretty soaps (in the shape of hearts, flowers, or even children's soaps shaped like teddy bears, lambs, or ducks) wrapped in net and tied with a ribbon
- High-quality wrapped chocolates or sugared almonds wrapped in fabric

- Box of animal crackers with string handle
- A cocktail umbrella with the guest's name written in calligraphy, placed on her plate
- Small decorative tin filled with nuts or sweets such as chocolate eggs

MENU

What are the traditional foods served at a baby shower?
Outside of a restaurant luncheon, it's best to keep the refreshments light and easy. Safe bets: a buffet of finger foods; passed-around hors d'oeuvres; tea and cookies; a buffet brunch with ready-to-serve foods, such as quiche, rolls, and fruit salad. No one expects a full sit-down meal at a baby shower. The centerpiece of the gathering is bestowing the presents on the mother, not carved meat and fancy soufflé. Showers are also uniquely convivial—put a dozen or more women in a room together focusing on babies, and you can count on plenty of clucking, reminiscing and advice-sharing. Guests want to circulate freely and gab.

Some communities follow the custom of a potluck shower. Unless you're sure this is the established mode among your friends, guests may not be too keen on it. In essence, you're asking them to bring two gifts: food and a baby present.

The guest of honor might be avoiding certain foods because she is pregnant. Do make a nonalcoholic punch or other festive fruit drink available (not eggnog). But avoid spiked punch, since it can be easily mistaken for punch without alcohol. It's okay to serve other alcoholic drinks, however, as well as coffee, tea, sodas: The pregnant woman has been used to avoiding these omnipresent beverages in others' company for months now. It's definitely thoughtful, however, to skip objectionable ingredients in the main course (such as sushi, sashimi) or the dessert (such as chocolate cake, if you know the mom-to-be has cut out chocolate).

Shower Refreshments

The following foods are easy to fix, serve, and eat in a party setting:

- Nonalcoholic fruit punch
- Spritzers (juice and sparkling water)
- Crudités and dip
- Crackers and cheese balls or dips
- Miniature individual quiches
- Finger sandwiches
- Hot hors d'oeuvres (stuffed mushrooms, kebabs, etc.)
- Chicken salad
- Casseroles
- Fruit salad (served in a watermelon cut and hollowed to look like a baby buggy)
- Fruit-and-yogurt parfaits
- Children's cookies: zwieback, animal crackers, wafer cookies, arrowroot biscuits
- Petit fours (or cake) decorated in keeping with your shower theme
- Angel food cake

IMPERFECT GIFTS

Can I return or exchange gifts I don't like?
What you do with the gifts you receive is your business. Baby-goods stores are used to returns and exchanges. Larger shops with vast inventories are even pretty good about trade-ins without a receipt. Your friends might wonder why they never see the outfit they provided or why the diaper stacker that clashes with your chosen nursery colors is not in use—but hopefully, they'll be too polite to ever mention the absence to you.

How do I handle duplicate gifts?
Thank the givers profusely. If the item is a piece of clothing, you can assure them that you love it so much that two of a kind are welcome. (Whether or not you decide to exchange one is up to you. If you really do adore it, consider trading one for a larger size.) If the item is obviously an unnecessary duplicate, such as a bathtub, one of the givers should offer to make the exchange or graciously say, "Of course you'll want to exchange that for something else. I bought it at XYZ Babyland, and I'm sure they'll take it back." If they both fail to speak up, however, just move on to the next gift after delivering your thanks. You neither need to dwell on the duplication at the shower—or tell them what you exchanged the gift for later.

RETURN GIFTS?

If there's a late miscarriage or stillbirth, should the shower presents be returned?

If a marriage were called off at the eleventh hour, the wedding presents would be returned. But the tragic loss of a much anticipated child is horrible for the parents to go through. Returning baby gifts might well be too painful, not to mention a low priority, for such a couple. If they want to send things back, that's fine. But if they don't, who could blame them? They could very properly store the gifts for possible future use, or donate them to charity.

THANK-YOUS

What's the statute of limitations on thank-you notes?
The customary interval for a response is within two to three weeks of receiving the gift. Smart moms-to-be put pen to paper right after the baby shower, since in the postpartum weeks they're too tired and too busy trying to keep up with all the additional congratulatory gifts that pour in. I attended one shower where the hostess passed around a guest book for guests to sign and provide their addresses. This was helpful because it was a gathering honoring a schoolteacher, and the guest list was a mix of her colleagues and her students' parents, so she may not have had everyone's addresses. (Only the honoree can write the actual notes.)

What if the months somehow slip by and your gifts go unthanked once your baby is not only sleeping through the night but taking her first steps? Write that note anyway. Better late than never. Enclose a cute baby picture to soften your faux pas.

Can I use note cards that have "thank you" preprinted on them?
Rigid manners mavens have always frowned on the practice. (You are supposed to write them on your personal notepaper.)

But it's the act of writing the note that's essential, not the paper you use. So long as you pen your own personal message inside such a card, it's not worth being a stickler over the sort of stationery. Your friends will be relieved to have any acknowledgment at all.

That said, if you care about the aesthetics of the deed, most blank notecards or stationery are a whole lot prettier or more interesting than the kind boringly stamped "thank you."

If someone gives money in lieu of a gift, should I refer to the exact amount in the thank-you note?
You can if you like, although it's not necessary. More importantly, you should let the giver know what you intend to spend the money on: "Thank you for the nice check. I am planning to use it toward a double stroller for the twins. As you might imagine, it's something we will really need."

How do I thank the people who throw my shower?
The mom-to-be should express her gratitude to the hosts who went to so much trouble with a note and a gift within a day or two of the event. Flowers are always a fitting gesture, as are a basket of soaps or lotions, homemade baked goods, or another personal token that you know the person will enjoy.

7

Naming the Baby

Making any kind of decision while you're pregnant can be difficult. Fortunately most choices are easily amended. Hate the Noah's Ark wallpaper you so lovingly selected? Redo it. Feel like a cow wearing that polka-dotted dress? Change it.

Naming your baby-to-be, on the other hand, is a more lasting decision. It affects not only you, but the person you wish the most for on the planet. Complicating matters, you're supposed to do it jointly with your partner. Everyone else you know may also render an opinion about this momentous responsibility—whether they're invited to or not.

It's little wonder most pregnant women begin obsessing about names soon after their pregnancy tests turn up positive. Your taste, your style, your capacity for teamwork, your very suitability as parents, all exposed in a few syllables! Or at least, that's how it can seem. Actually, naming a baby is a wonderful opportunity, one of the most special things about pregnancy. It's your first gift to your baby.

CONVENTIONS

What should be considered in choosing a name?
Above all, select a name that you like. You'll have used it about a million times by the time your baby leaves home.

You will coo it. You whisper it. You will yell it. You will make funny nicknames out of it.

Take care that the name sounds good (admittedly a subjective thing). Say it aloud with the last name (surname) and in a combination with possible middle names.

Not least, think of your child. He or she is the one who will bear the name throughout life. A good name transcends fashion or a parent's fancy, spares the child embarrassment or confusion, and is something the child will wear with pride on his or her life's journey. A name with special significance or meaning is icing on the cake that may spur your child to greater things. Some researchers believe that one's name is one's destiny—your name can influence your future success, social acceptance, and psychological well-being!

What cultural traditions might govern the name selection?
Parents seeking a name that has personal meaning can turn to their ancestry for inspiration. Many excellent baby-name guides are now available for particular ethnic or religious persuasions; ask at any good bookstore or library. Here are some general cultural practices:

African-American customs

The use of African names has seen a rebirth in the past twenty years as African-Americans celebrate their cultural heritage. Some parents feel that bestowing an African name helps to connect a child to his or her past in a way that a European name can't.

Traditionally, a great deal of consideration is given to the name's meaning. For example, African names often describe a characteristic or trait. Dara means "elegant" in Yoruba, and Marini is Swahili for "fresh, healthy, and pretty." The name may also reflect a wish for the child, such as Nyoka, Swahili for "be honest." Other names describe a circumstance of the birth. Example: Pacha is Zulu for "one of twins." Damina means "rainy season" in Hausa, a Nigerian language, and Daren is Hausa for "born at night." Names also come from the spiritual realm, such as "Cis" from the Ibo god Chi. Most African names are genderless, although some may have a more masculine or a more feminine ring to modern American ears.

Another trend is to mine black history for worthy role-model names. Examples: Rosa (Parks); Thurgood (Marshall); Zora (Neale Hurston); Langston (Hughes). African history reveals inspiring names as well, such as Candace (used by five Ethopian queens) or Ashanti (an ancient kingdom that was an art center). Bestowing a name with historic or cultural meaning gives you an opportunity to educate your child about this very personal source of self-esteem as he or she grows up.

Another African-American fashion is to use names that are neither European nor African. These made-up monikers rely more on creative license than factual heritage. For example, new names are often created by adding an extra syllable to the beginning or end of a common name: Lasue (from Sue); Dejay (from Jay), Annre (from Ann), Donell (from Don). Fresh names are also created by changing letters in traditional names. Examples: Dvonne (from Yvonne) or Nishelle (from Michelle).

Some African-influenced names are more common or easier to spell and pronounce than others. Parents selecting them need to weigh the benefits of self-image and cultural pride against potential confusion or even discrimination that a child may encounter as the result of an unusual name. Some parents balance the first and middle name so that if one is unique, the other is not.

Catholic customs

The name of a Catholic saint is traditionally given for a child's first or middle name. It's hoped that the namesake may imitate his or her patron's saintly virtues, pray to him or her for guidance, and that the saint will help to watch over the child in heaven. Parents therefore educate their child about the saint's life as he or she grows up. Naming a child after a saint is no longer a requirement of the church, though a saint's name or one with Christian significance is still recommended. (*Exception:* The name Jesus is frowned on in America, considered too holy for common usage. On the other hand, it is common in Spanish-speaking Catholic countries.)

Some children are named with the traits or story of a particular saint in mind. St. George, for example, was a Roman soldier known for his boldness and bravery, who died for his faith. St. Francis of Assisi was a great lover of nature. Others are named for the saint whose feast day it is on the day of the baby's birth. For example, January 26 is the feast day of St. Paula, who died on that date. St. Sylvester, a former pope, has the date December 31. The church publishes an annual calendar of feast days; it's also posted on the web at *http://saints.catholic.org*. In many Catholic countries, one's saint's feast day is celebrated with as much fanfare as the American birthday.

Another variation is to name your child after the patron saint of one of your hobbies, occupations, or favorite places. Therese of Lisieux is one of the patron saints of flower-lovers and growers, for example. Gregory the Great is the patron saint of teachers. Maybe you'd like to commemorate your honeymoon in Paris (where the patron saint is Genevieve) or Venice (Mark) or Sweden (Bridget).

Japanese customs

Names are chosen that will render good luck on the child. Therefore, special attention is given to the name's meaning. Common examples: Hideo ("excellent boy"); Hideaki ("smart one"), Kei ("respect"); Koko ("stork," a symbol of longevity); Tomiko ("contented"). Many names conjure virtuous natural images: Yuki ("snow"); Sakura ("cherry blossom," a symbol of prosperity).

It's also considered fortuitous to name a child after a rounded number. The girl's name Yachiko, for example, means "eight thousand." Numbers may also reflect birth order: Taro ("firstborn son"), Jiro ("second son").

Jewish customs

American Jews commonly name their child in honor of an ancestor of the same sex. Typically two names are selected: one Hebrew name that is used for religious occasions (such as Herschel, after Great-uncle Herschel) and a secular name that begins with the same letter, by which the child will commonly be known (such as Harrison). Sometimes the Hebrew name merely shares the same first initial, for example Hillel, in honor of Great-uncle Herschel, though the child is called Harrison.

Variations: You might choose to give the baby just one name (such as Ruth, after Great-aunt Ruth). Or use the relative's Hebrew name as a middle name combined with a secular first name (such as Jessica Devorah for Grandma Devorah). Also consider the name's meaning. Mildred, for example, means "gentle strength." An equivalent Hebrew name would be Gabrielle ("God is my strength").

It is also possible to name your child after an ancestor of the opposite sex.

Most American Jews name their children only after deceased ancestors, in keeping with Ashkenazic (middle-European) tradition. To name an infant after a living person, tradition goes, would rob that person of his or her full life. Sephardic Jews (of the Middle East and elsewhere), however, do give the names of living relatives or friends.

Traditional biblical names—Benjamin, Adam, Hanna, Abigail—are making a comeback. Another trend is to address the child throughout life by his or her traditional Hebrew name: Shoshana, Tivona, Tobit, Avram, Gideon, Shayna. Names that are rarely used by Jewish families include Natalie and Noel (Christmas), Christopher (one who carries Christ), and Dolores (sorrow of the Virgin Mary).

Muslim customs

Generally traditional names are preferred. Often they are the names of the descendants of the Prophet Muhammad and his family, such as Ali, Ayasha, Hinda. The name Muhammad itself has hundreds of popular variations: Mahmud; Amed; Ahmad; Hamid; and Hamdun are but a few.

Names that reference a virtue are also favored. Examples: Sharif ("honest"); Yasar ("wealth"), Amineh ("faithful"). Popular names of Arabic origin reflect the ninety-nine qualities of God as described in the Qu'ran. Examples: Hakeem ("wise"); Karim ("generous"), Kamil ("perfect").

Native American customs

A name is believed to be very personal, akin to one's very soul. Because names are so individual, a child is rarely given a parent's or other relative's name. Rather, American Indian monikers often describe natural phenomenon or the circumstances at birth. Examples: Pukuna (Miwok for "deer jumping downhill"); Tadi (Omaha for "wind"); Huyana (Miwok for "rain falling").

Names may also describe a characteristic, such as Wapi ("lucky"); Yuma ("son of the chief"), Lenmana ("flute maiden"). Given the infinite variety of possibilities, there are relatively few "common" Native American names. Some names have Spanish influences, such as Ninita, used by the Zuni.

Puerto Rican customs

A firstborn child is frequently named after the parent or god-parent of the same sex. Godparents are highly esteemed among Catholic Puerto Ricans. Diminutives are also common. For example, the godmother may be Carmen, and the baby is known as Carmencita ("little Carmen"). Diminutives of the popular name Francisco include those as different-sounding as Chico, Pancho, and Paquito.

Many girls' names reflect homage to the Virgin Mary. These include not only the popular Maria (often blended with a middle name, such as Maria Elena, Maria Concetta) but also Luz ("Light"), Jesusa ("Mary of Jesus"), and Pilar ("pillar," since Mary is a pillar of the Catholic faith). This tradition is true in other Spanish-speaking Catholic countries as well.

Other customs

Ask family members on both sides what customs are common in your clan. Many Italians, for example, traditionally name the firstborn son after the paternal grandfather and the first-born daughter after the paternal grandmother. The second-borns of each gender are named after the maternal grandparents. It's a custom in Denmark and other countries to honor a beloved relative with a namesake, even if others in the extended family have already used the identical name for their children.

Sources of Inspiration

Can't decide? Brainstorming sources are literally all around you. You may not want to admit that your baby's name came from a favorite soap opera or the latest bodice-ripper you've read, but then again, it's nobody's business exactly how you arrived at your choice. (If your chosen name really did come from a soap, do your child a favor and never admit it.)

More places to look:

- Your family tree
- Friends or relatives you admire
- Baby-name guides (Don't overlook specialty guides to ethnic names. Or you can select a name based on the original meaning of the word or one of its variations.)
- History books, for noteworthy figures
- The dictionary
- A map or atlas
- The Bible, Torah, or Qu'ran
- Pregnancy and parenting web sites (many offer name inventories)
- Baby-naming computer software programs
- Your parents' or grandparents' high-school yearbooks (for oldies that sound new again)
- Your local newspaper's birth announcement listings
- Favorite works of literature (authors or characters)

- The telephone directory
- Your own names (Joe + Elizabeth = JoBeth; Barbara + Larry = Barry; my daughter Page's name is a hybrid of Paula and George.)

JUNIOR

When can "junior" be used after a name?
Only a boy who is named exactly the same as his father is properly called "junior." The suffix "Jr." (always capitalized when abbreviated, or written out in lowercase) appears after his name. The father then becomes "senior" (or "Sr."). The father's suffix is not normally used, however, even when the name appears in print. It's mostly a conversational distinction used when describing the two different individuals.

Example: When President John Fitzgerald Kennedy named his son after himself, the boy was properly called John Fitzgerald Kennedy, Jr. The president officially became "John Fitzgerald Kennedy, Sr." although that title was not used in writing. Traditionally, the "junior" is dropped when the father dies. Upon President Kennedy's death, his son became "John Fitzgerald Kennedy." (The press persisted in referring to him as "JFK, Jr." in order to distinguish the two famous men.)

When both grandfather and father are still alive (if they have identical names), the newborn becomes "the third" (written as 3rd or in Roman numerals as III.) Normally such numerical titles are dropped as the senior relatives die. When a grandfather who held the title "Sr." passes away, his son (the former "Jr.") becomes "senior" and his grandson (formerly, "3rd") becomes "Jr." That's why you don't hear about very many "sevenths" and "eighths." (Except in the British royal family, where the numerals assigned to British kings and queens have historic purposes; therefore, their rules—no pun intended—don't apply to we commoners.)

Exception: When family names are carried across several generations, the subsequent name changes following a relative's death can be confusing for the individuals affected and their acquaintances—not to mention their legal and business records. Therefore, some men elect to retain their suffixes even after the elder relations pass away. Sometimes a suffix inspires a nickname to distinguish the generations. For example, Microsoft's Bill Gates (William H. Gates III) is called Trey by his father, William H. Gates, Jr.

Then there's George Foreman, the boxer, who named all four of his sons George: George, Jr., George III, George IV, and George V. He also has daughters named Georgetta and Freeda George.

What's the difference between calling your child a "junior" or "the second"?
The only time "the second" is used is when a boy is given exactly the same name as another living relative, other than his father. If Mr. and Mrs. Ethan Allen Smith decide to name their son after his uncle Thomas Jones Smith, the child becomes Thomas Jones Smith, 2nd (or II). When the senior relative dies, however, the namesake drops the numerals after his name.

What do you call a son who is named after his father, but who is not the firstborn son?
A boy whose name is identical to his father uses the suffix "Jr." whether he is the first son or the fifth. Therefore if Ethan Allen Smith names his firstborn Thomas Jones Smith and chooses to name his next son after himself, that boy is "Ethan Allen Smith, Jr." He is not "Ethan Allen Smith, II." There's no rule that says only the first son is eligible to be a namesake.

Can a child be called "Jr." if his middle name differs from his father's, or if he has an extra name?

No. Only a son whose name is identical to his father's may properly have the suffix "Jr." added to his name. President George Herbert Walker Bush's son, the Texas governor, is also a George Bush, but not a George Bush, Jr. That's because his full name is George Walker Bush—no Herbert.

Is a girl named after her mother called "Jr."?

Baby girls used to be named after their mothers far more commonly than is done today. But even when the names are identical, the custom of adding the suffix "Jr." or "second" after a name is reserved for males. The reason is that names are traditionally handed down according to the male branches of a family tree.

Exception: A woman who is married to a "junior" can use that suffix when it's attached to her husband's name, as in "Mrs. Cal Ripken, Jr." But this little anachronism is rarely used anymore, since most women prefer to go by their own first names, rather than their husband's. It is not proper, however, for a woman married to a junior to use her first name with the suffix, as in "Mrs. Kelly Ripken, Jr."

MIDDLE NAMES

How many middle names can be used?

As many as you like. Middle names are a relatively recent phenomenon, which began as the population grew, to help distinguish between *this* John the Wheelwright and *that* John the Wheelwright. Initially, middle names tended to be the mother's maiden name. In the seventeenth century, giving more than one Christian name gained popularity in England and France after the daughters of Charles II were christened

Charlotte Jemima and Henrietta Maria. By the eighteenth century, it was common for girls, especially, to receive three or more names. These were often inspired by relatives, god-parents, and works of romantic literature.

Most people today opt for one middle name. Some children, particularly in the South, are called by both names: Ruth Ellen, Billy Ray, Laura Lee, James Earl. It's also common for children to be known familiarly only by their middle names, rather than their given names. If both father and son are named John, for example, but with different middle names, the son may be called by his middle name to distinguish him.

Some parents select the order of names according to how they sound. They may even then prefer to use the name that falls in the middle. So they name their daughter "Anastasia May," but call her "May." While melodic, this practice is somewhat confusing all around.

Many families give multiple middle names. When Diana Spencer married Prince Charles in 1981, who could blame her for stumbling over his name—Charles Philip Arthur George—as they exchanged vows? Some couples insert the mother's maiden name (or her surname, if she did not change it when she married) as one of the baby's middle names, along with two Christian names.

Stringing lots of names together is a handy way to pacify interested relatives. On the other hand, you might find it cumbersome, and you (or, eventually, your child) probably won't be able to include all the names when filling out various forms down the line. A British gentleman in the nineteenth century reportedly named his daughter Anna Bertha Cecilia Diana Emily Fanny Gertrude Hypatia Inez Jane Kate Louisa Maud Nora Ophelia Quince Rebecca Sarah Teresa Ulysses Venus Winifred Xenophon Yetty Zeus. (Surname: Pepper.) President Harry Truman's parents simply chose "S," which didn't actually stand for anything, although it indirectly honored both of their fathers, Solomon and Shipp. Some families don't select any middle name at all—though this seems a little stingy.

Some options for middle names:

- Another name you like
- The mother's maiden name (or surname)
- The name of a relative, friend, or public figure you wish to honor (first name or surname)
- The name of a relative on the opposite side of the family, if the first name comes from one side
- A significant day or season, or a related word (such as Noelle for a Christmas baby or Millie for a girl born in 2000)
- A personality trait you wish to bestow (such as Patience)
- A place name of significance (provided it has the melodic ring of a name, not "Hoboken" or "Sneedville")

It is true that when family names are used, the first name ought to come from one side of the family and the middle name ought to come from the other parent's side?
This is a family convention for some, rather than a formal rule. Tit-for-that naming can be an equitable way of eking out a compromise. Variation: Some couples agree to let one parent select the first name while the other parent chooses the second.

Should I still use a middle name if my child will also have both my surname and his father's—that would make four names?
If you want to. It depends on your appetite for lengthy appellations. Many women who retain their maiden names after

marriage choose to incorporate that name into their baby's. If you also choose a second middle name, this makes for a lengthy full name that defies many forms and may not actually be used by the child through school.

A simpler option would be to use the maiden name as the middle name. This, however, deprives the parents of the fun of selecting two names.

More Naming Traditions

- A British superstition warns against giving your child a name once used by a family pet.
- Sephardic Jewish grandparents consider it a blessing to have many children named after them during their lifetime.
- The ancient Romans often numbered their children: Primus, Secundus, Tertius (First, Second, Third), or for girls, Prima, Secunda, Tertia.
- It's a Hawaiian tradition to dream a name. The content of your dreams is said to reveal clues and symbols.
- The Puritans liked to invent names, usually rooted in Christian virtues (Charity, Humility) or biblical goals (Increase, Treadwell).
- A Scandinavian custom calls for the parents to stencil the baby's name or initials on the wall above his or her sleeping place.
- Many cultures give a baby a public "false name" to trick evil spirits until an official naming ceremony is held.
- Victorians did not speak the child's name until the christening.

> • In Uganda, Lango babies are told a series of names while they are offered the breast. They receive the name spoken when they begin to nurse.

SURNAMES

What are our options for the baby's surname if the parents' names are different?
The simplest, and most traditional, thing to do is to give the newborn the father's last name, whether the parents are married or not.

Exceptions abound, especially in the last twenty-five years. Some families create a whole new surname for their clan. This can be done through hyphenation, so that Mary Smith and Tom Jones have a baby named Sue Ellen Smith-Jones. (Mary and Tom could both change their surnames to Smith-Jones as well.) Or it can be done with more creative twists: Ann Foster and Jacob Hellbender naming their baby Timothy Fosbender. In one family where the parents had different surnames, they gave their firstborn the father's last name and the next child the mother's. (They did not have a tiebreaker third.) Another family used the mother's last name for the girls and the father's for the boys.

Such variations foster egalitarianism, make a point for feminism, and perhaps accomplish other worthy aims. But if you're uncertain, let me be one small voice in favor of patriarchy, at least regarding family names. An entire family who shares the same surname spares others confusion and underscores unity. Avoiding hyphens ensures a simpler future, when Sue Ellen Smith-Jones marries Ronald Parker-Moniker. Not least, traditional surnames make research much easier on future generations trying to retrace their family tree.

What last name should a single mother use for her baby when the father is not in the picture?
Traditionally babies or unwed parents are given the father's surname. But when the father is not going to be part of his child's life, it may be more comfortable for the child as he or she grows if the child's last name is the same as the mother's.

TELLING OTHERS

What's the best way to respond to people who ask if we've picked out a name and we have, but don't want to tell?
To say, "We know but we're keeping it a secret" is teasing. You'll be besieged by begs for hints or goaded into divulging the information: "Come on, you can tell me. I'm your sister. I won't tell a soul!"

Far simpler to tell a little white social lie: "We're still thinking about it." This spares you the goading as well as the unwelcome opinions that are inevitably leveled against a name that has been announced but not yet attached to a breathing human being. Also, even if you've decided, you might change your mind. One look at little John in the delivery room, and you might be struck by what a Paul he really is. Or a George. Or a Ringo. If you've already insisted to everyone that you're expecting a John, you might wind up with monogrammed blankets and engraved silver cups that are now all wrong.

WHEN PARTNERS DISAGREE

How can partners reach a compromise?
Compromise is the operative word here. Choosing a name that satisfies both parents is all about give-and-take. Inevi-

tably, your partner will have had a horrid college roommate with the very name you love, or your favorites will remind your mate of an unpleasant movie character, until you cancel one another out so many times that you feel sure you've gone through every possibility. Take a deep breath. A name is important, but it's only a name. If you think this is hard, just wait until you're wrangling over discipline in a few years.

Now get hold of one of those books promising 5,000 or 10,000 or 100,000 great baby names, and follow these suggestions:

- *Make it clear up front which things are most important to you in a name.* One woman had a family tradition, stretching back five generations, that the firstborn daughter was always named Mary (each with a different middle name, by which she was commonly known). Italian and Greek families often name children after relatives in a prescribed order, such as the first son after the father's father; the second son after the mother's father, and so on. Maybe the name's meaning is paramount to one parent. (For my own husband, one of the ground rules was that he was not going to pick his children's names out of a book.)
- *Draw up top ten lists.* Each of you comes up with ten (or twenty) names that you could live with. Exchange lists and see if there are any matches. If not, go back to the drawing board.
- *Avoid outside influences.* If you're really having trouble, try not to enlist other friends or relatives to your "side" to mount a campaign for a particular moniker. Anyway, the more opinions you hear, the more confused you're liable to feel. Keep it private.
- *Say the name out loud.* Hearing it (with your last name)

may sound better than simply reading it. Also remember that babies grow into their names. "Benjamin" or "Lucinda" may seem big on a newborn, but newborns grow.

- *Stay neutral.* Before dismissing a name outright that your partner is very fond of, first try to live with it for a few days or weeks. Then render your opinion. Also avoid joking and whining.

- *Split the task.* Once you agree on a first name that was offered by one partner, let the other partner select the middle name (perhaps from a short list of possibilities you both agree on). Or if one person chooses the name, the other could decide on the spelling (Catherine with a C or with a K?).

NAMESAKES

Should you ask permission to name your child after someone?
Making your child the namesake of a beloved family member, a good friend, your family doctor, or another living person is bestowing an honor on that person. It's not necessary to ask first if you may do so. The individual ought to be flattered. And if he (or she) is not, he should keep that opinion to himself.

Does someone who has a child named after them have special obligations to that child?
No. Having a namesake is not the same as being a godparent, or even an aunt or an uncle. It's natural to take a continued special interest in the child who shares your name, but you don't "owe" him or her anything.

How do you let it be known that you *haven't* named your baby after someone, that it was just a coincidence that the names are the same?

What if, for example, your beloved aunt and your loathed boss share the same first name? All you need to say, when colleagues remark on the name or on the coincidence, is that you christened your child after her Great-aunt Marguerite. You cannot tell your boss, "Sorry, but you're not the Marguerite we had in mind." You can, however, say, "I knew you would like it. It's an old family name. I always promised my favorite aunt that I would name my first daughter after her."

NICKNAMES

How do we make clear that we plan to use the formal name, not a nickname version?

By using that name. My firstborn son is named Henry. When he was born, coworkers and friends continually asked me how "little Hank" was doing. Never mind that "Henry" and "Hank" don't even sound alike, and that his birth announcement read "Henry," and that that's the only way my husband and I ever referred to him. So I would simply reply that "Henry is doing fine." (Gentle accent on the first word.)

When your child is in day care or begins school, ask his caregivers and teachers to use the proper name, too. Eventually everyone should catch on—including your child. (When my son, now seven, is referred to as "Hank," he simply looks blank.) Once your child's peers get hold of him, however, it may be a different story. Unless *he's* the one who insists on being called Lawrence or Charles or Henry, you may wind up with a Larry or Chuck or Hank after all.

One bright note: Things may be easier today than if you tried bestowing a traditional moniker back in the sixties, seventies and early eighties, when clipped names (Tom, Sue) and those ending in a chummy "y" (Billy, Sally) were the rage. Kids are now growing up with classes full of Jonathons and Elizabeths, who are far less likely to be turned into Johnnys and Bettys.

UNUSUAL NAMES

How far can we go in creating a special name for our child? Certainly all bursting-with-pride parents think their babies are special and deserve the best—starting with a special name. After all, names are deeply personal matters into which a great deal of thought and love are usually given. Whatever the choice, it's just not polite to poke fun. But remember that choosing a name is one of the first major decisions you'll make on behalf of your child, a responsibility that he will bear the results of his entire life—or until he's old enough to legally amend it, should he despise it. Finding a name that is special is admirable; finding one that is unique can be dicey. There's a fine line between individual and indigestible.

Oddness is in the eye of the bestower, but there's plenty to consider. It's become popular, for example, to give a traditional name the twist of an atypical spelling. The idea, in theory, is for the child to feel of the mainstream, yet with a dollop of individual flair. Thus we have Jaymz, Zakery, Brittenee, Meegin, Jazminn, et. al. Do you really want your child to spend his whole life correcting others on the spelling of his name? Or worse, having his name look like an error whenever seen in print?

Really corny names hit their zenith (or nadir) in the 1960s: Moonbeam, Sunshine, Free Bird, Mountain, Zen, et. al. The conspicuous consumption-crazed eighties and nineties saw their own flurry of made-up names of dubious taste. Babies were named after cars (Miata, Lexus, Porsche); department stores (Bloomingdale, Macy, Tiffany); and other forms of prestige (Cashmere, Yale, Chanel). Who knows what the twenty-first century will bring? John.com? E-mily? R*lph? Whether you lead the way is up to you.

FIRST DIBS

What if we want to use a name that a relative has already said that she prefers?
First consider the extenuating circumstances: Is this relative pregnant? Is she even married yet? What's so special about this name? If she isn't pregnant (or married), why is she going around telling people what she plans to name her hypothetical child?

A name is a very personal thing, and many people view them a bit like private property. They're not, however, even when attached to a living breathing human. Names are a first-come, first-served commodity. If a relative chooses a name you like for her child who is born before yours, it's your prerogative to either go ahead with your plans to use it, or to come up with another favorite. Ditto if you should happen to preempt someone else. It's courteous (and eventually less confusing) to choose an alternative—or at least use a different nickname—if a close family member has beaten you to the punch. But there's nothing inappropriate about a pair of cousins sharing one name. As one woman who made her child a relative's second namesake explained, "Aunt Pamela was so special and worthy, we decided there was enough honor to go around."

Take the Name Test

Before you settle on a name, ask yourselves the following questions. (There are no right or wrong answers, but the way you feel about some of your responses may lead you to second-guess a potentially troublesome name.)

- Is the name easy to pronounce? Straightforward pronunciations will spare your child a certain amount of embarrassment and constant correcting of others.
- Is it easy to say? Consider the number of syllables in each name and where their accents fall. Do they flow or sound jarring? Typically a long surname works best with a short first name, and vice versa: George Washington, Virginia Woolf.
- Is it easy to spell? Sure, switching out a "y" for an "i" puts an individual stamp on the name. It may also condemn your child to a lifetime of misspelled mail, hassles with the IRS, and confusion with people taking orders by phone.
- Do the child's initials spell an unfortunate word or acronym? (For example, DUD, UFO, SAP, JERK)? Also check the monogram, which usually reads first name–surname–middle name.
- Does the name have any common nicknames that you cannot abide? You may not be able to control what peers call your child down the road. (Consistent usage will give your preferred name an edge, but there are no guarantees.)

- How will the name sound on top of a resume? As a CEO? When yelled out the back door at suppertime? Consider its usage throughout the child's life.
- Is it a unisex name and if so, does this bother you? Many boys' names have been so frequently given to girls that they no longer sound masculine to modern ears (Ashley, Leslie, Kelly, Lynn). Other names are routinely used by both sexes, which may set the child up for some confusion later in life (Dakota, Alex, Taylor, Drew).
- If it's a trendy name, will it bother you to find five other Michaelas or Noahs in your child's kindergarten class? Consult most-popular-baby-name guides to evaluate just how unique your favorite choices really are.
- Do both parents agree on it?
- Do you like it? You'll be living with it for a long time.

CRITICISM

What's the right response to someone who criticizes or ridicules our chosen name?
You certainly owe no apologies or defenses. To have your choice be damned by anyone is insulting and out of line. Frown slightly, and say, "I'm sorry you feel that way. I hope you'll learn to like it as Chynestra grows into it." The last thing you want to do is get into a debate with this person on the merits of *their* ideas on the subject.

Beware that most people tend to be more freely critical of names learned before the baby's birth. It may be that the baby seems more abstract to them, and therefore the name does, too. Before birth, many people may not even realize that they are being rude in commenting on your selection. The other party may also feel that expectant parents are more vulnerable to influence or persuasion before the birth.

INDECISION

Must we settle on a name before we leave the hospital?
It's not strictly necessary. Some couples have waited weeks (to their relatives' consternation). "It does raise eyebrows to leave the hospital without a name," says one mom who waited eight days before settling on "Katheryn Grace." "And it can be stressful if you're worried what other people think, or if you're worried about disappointing your husband, like I was," she adds. "On the other hand, why not take time, if you need it, to get the name you love?"

Even this woman advises others of the benefits to getting this little detail out of the way before you're admitted to the hospital. You do have some nine months to work on the problem, and only need to come up with two possibilities. (Unless you've had amnio or CVS and are genetically positive of the gender—ultrasound being notoriously imperfect—it's smart to have two names just in case.) Once the baby arrives there are too many other things to think about, like how you're going to get some sleep and how to soothe your sore nipples.

You may also be charged a late fee if you do not supply a name at the time the birth certificate is filed in the hospital.

What do we do if we change our minds about the baby's name?
It can be costly and confusing to alter a newborn's name after the birth certificate has been filed. Many states levy a charge to make any change, even if to correct a typo or other mistake. For this reason it's important to review the forms for

the birth certificate very carefully while you are in the hospital.

Ten Things One Never Should Say About a Baby's Name

- "Oh everybody has that name."
- "Gee, I've never heard a name like that."
- "I've always hated that name."
- "Where did you come up with that one?"
- "I know someone awful who has that name (but I'm sure your baby will be different)."
- "Isn't that a little trendy?"
- "Isn't that a little old-fashioned?"
- "What's wrong with my name?"
- "What's wrong with Grandpa's/Grandma's/his father's name?"
- "Is it too late to change your mind?"

8

Birth

*T*he big day! Surely a woman so great with child has more things on her mind than manners. Etiquette ought to be the last thing on your mind in the middle of a C-section. No one expects you to greet a single nurse with a handshake and a "How do you do?"

Still, there are some issues of propriety to be considered about the day your baby's born, from who's present at the birth to how people are told about it afterward. Many customs and traditions can also help to shape the birth experience.

The baby may be the star, but there are plenty of other people to consider also on this most magical day.

ATTENDEES

How do I tell eager friends and family that I don't want them present at the birth?

You don't have to say anything. A birth is not an event to which anyone ought to expect an invitation, much less be disinvited from. It's almost hard to imagine that just ten or fifteen years ago, a birth was considered a private event for the parents only. And just fifteen or twenty years before that, not even the father was welcome!

Should someone you know appear to be angling for an

invitation—or worse, simply assume that they'll be welcome—you may need to be more firm. Say something like, "I know that Pam and Sam invited you to their baby's birth, but Joe and I are planning a more private delivery. We'll call you as soon as the baby's here."

Some hospitals allow you to place limits on visitors, including who may be present during delivery and who may visit during specific hours afterward.

What do I do if I want my parents present, but they don't like the idea?

Some couples like the idea of sharing the wonder of birth with other people they love. The degree of privacy one craves at this intimate time is a matter of personal taste.

Some grandmothers-to-be embrace such an opportunity, particularly if they were not very active participants in their own deliveries, as was common through the late seventies, or if they had C-sections. But others—and many granddads-to-be—may be understandably squeamish about the notion. Or there may be other reasons they do not wish to be present, such as believing that the birth should be a special time between you and your partner. Perhaps they have a concern, sometimes legitimate, that their presence may detract from your ability to relax and concentrate during contractions. Even if you're convinced that they would cherish the experience, all you can do is extend the invitation. You can't force them to come, after all. Nor should you hold it against them if they decline the chance. You can bet they'll rush to meet their new grandbaby afterward ASAP.

Should children witness birth?

This is more of a question of psychology than etiquette. Expert opinions are sharply divided. In one camp fall those who feel that witnessing a mother crying out in pain can be distressful for a young sibling. The mother's ability to focus on labor may be impaired. Proponents of the practice feel that witnessing birth is a learning experience that can draw children closer to their parents and to their new sibling.

Consider the age of the child. A toddler or young preschooler will not understand the mechanics of birth, even with preparation. A young child will have a hard time understanding why Mommy and Daddy can't attend to his or her needs right away. If the delivery is in a hospital, the medical equipment may be frightening. The child may simply get bored.

An older child should be prepared in advance about what will happen, perhaps by watching videos about birth or attending prenatal visits, to reduce feelings of fear or confusion. Whatever the child's age, there should be a baby-sitter present whose sole job is to look after the child. This is a good idea even when the birth is at home. Neither parent can realistically expect to fulfill this role.

BIRTH PARTY

What is a birth party and how are invitations issued?
Increasingly, couples are viewing birth as a cause for celebration—from the moment the child takes the first breath, or sooner. They're inviting family and friends to gather 'round right in the delivery room.

The rise of the private birthing room at maternity centers and hospitals has contributed to the trend, as has standard usage of the epidural, which minimizes labor's misery for Mom.

"Guests" are invited verbally. Obviously, they can't RSVP,

since they can't usually know in advance when the blessed event will occur. They often arrive with champagne and hors d'oeuvres. There may be music, too.

Whether this current vogue is a good idea depends on your appetite for large numbers of people staring into your privates and egging you on through contractions. (Your father? Your grandfather? Your cousin? Your neighbor?) Some families are more communal than others. What is comforting and relaxing to one laboring woman may be irritating to another.

First-time parents are at the disadvantage of not knowing what birth will be like or how they will react to it. Some women retreat to a primal state in labor, and greatly prefer to be alone. Even if the parents decide on a birth party for their delivery, the mother reserves the right to shoo everyone out of the room if she changes her mind midstream. Participants must also be prepared to leave in the event of a medical emergency.

If the group-birth idea appeals to you, be sure you have the okay of your birthing center in advance. There may be a limit on the number of people who may be in your room at one time, or restrictions on children's ages. Or you could plan on a home birth.

LABOR SUPPORT

Does my partner have to be my labor coach?
No. Many men are terrific at it, but not all. They baby's father serving as labor support person is a strictly late-twentieth-century invention. The role inspires excitement and confidence in some couples, and panic in others. Rightly so. The truth is, you can be a great father but a lousy labor coach. Some men are squeamish. They may worry that they won't

be able to read their wife's signals and help her accordingly. They may feel helpless, or distressed to see her in pain.

If the father does not want to serve as labor supporter—or if the mother doesn't want him to—neither party should feel bad. What's important is that the couple try to plan an optimal birth experience. An alternative to dad is to enlist a friend or relative (such as a sister or a mother), who would attend childbirth-preparation classes with the couple.

Or you can hire a professional labor supporter. The use of a labor *doula* (from the Greek word for handmaiden) is growing rapidly. These women are trained in the process of labor and in how to provide physical and emotional comfort. It's an art, not an instinct that all of us are born with. Whereas the doctor or midwife is chiefly concerned with the woman's and baby's physical progress, the doula is there to lend emotional support. Research shows that labors are shorter and less complicated in the presence of a doula, and the likelihood of using epidural anesthetic is reduced by more than half.

Just because a dad-to-be is not going to assume the primary labor support role doesn't mean he is superfluous, though. Far from it. A partner's presence can be a calming influence on a laboring woman, even if he is simply sitting in the room or having half-moons gouged in his hand by his wife's clutching fingernails.

Can others in the birthing room watch TV or listen to the radio?

If the laboring mother finds music soothing, as many do, she ought to have it. Ditto television, although it's a rare woman who can concentrate on the plot of *The X-Files* during contractions. A far more common occurrence, however, is for the dad-to-be to turn on a ball game during the delivery. This is a big no-no.

Why shouldn't he tune in, since he's just waiting around anyway? Here's why: He should not watch TV because he is not just waiting for a pizza to be delivered. He is waiting for the birth of his child, which is one of life's most momentous experiences. Besides that, his partner may need him to mop her brow or fetch her ice chips. For anyone present in the delivery room to act like anything is more important than the big woman lying there moaning is worse than rude, it's inhumane.

How does one ask a friend to be a labor coach, and what are her obligations?

Since this is a role you should reserve for your nearest and dearest—not to mention your most reliable—friend, all you need to do is blurt the question out. Do so early in pregnancy, so she can think it over and to give you time to find a replacement if she's unable to fill the job.

Your labor-support person should attend all childbirth-preparation classes with you, and tour the place where you will deliver. She (or he) may also attend some prenatal visits. As your due date nears, the person should be in constant easy contact, even if it means renting a pager for a few weeks. She ought to help you get to the hospital or birthing center, if the baby's father is unable to do so, and stay at your side until the baby is born. Once a labor-supporter has agreed to perform the job, there's no backing out. Be sure the individual doesn't have unexpected travel assignments at work or other responsibilities that might prevent him or her from coming through when it counts.

OUT OF CONTROL

If I do or say something embarrassing or unkind in labor, must I apologize after?
Just as a natural amnesia develops after birth, clouding a mother's memory of the intensity of her labor pain, so too should she—and everybody else who was present—forget anything that she said or did during the experience. Women have been known to swear at, insult, hit, scratch, throw up on, and otherwise abuse their mates or the hospital staff while in the throes of labor. Suffice it to say that one is not entirely one's normal self during delivery. And so the normal rules of conduct are suspended, for a bit.

Needless to say, offended parties must let the remarks and actions pass without negative comment. This is hardly a time to pick a fight.

A mother who's later mortified by some fuzzy memory can smile weakly, and say, "Sorry if I wasn't my usual self there" or "I hope I didn't cause you too much trouble." And then both parties should best let it go at that.

No loving partner should hold a grudge or tell tales on the new mother.

FILMING BIRTH

Is videotaping a birth in good taste?
It's not the filming itself that's questionable, it's what's being shot and how it's done. Many large hospitals have an outright ban on video equipment, out of fear of malpractice lawsuits. This is a shame. Many parents like this live-action memento of their child's first breath. (Although to whom it's properly

shown later is another matter.) One large study of Iowa doctors found that videotaping can be a positive thing all around, when doctors and patients agree on its use.

Find out your doctor's preferences in advance. A consent form signed by both parties may remove any legal issues. It should cover such matters as getting the mother's consent in writing and agreeing to stop recording if there are complications.

In the delivery room, the taper should use discretion. Position the camera from the mother's head or at her side, so that the miraculous moment of birth is clearly visible but not unnecessarily graphic. A tripod is a good idea because it can be set up out of everyone's way, and free the father for more important tasks—like being at his wife's side.

Videotaping a birth is not considerate when:

- The mother does not want to be filmed
- The mother's request to avoid direct shots of her vagina are ignored
- The taper is intruding in the doctors' and nurses' space and making it difficult for them to do their jobs
- The taper is physically or verbally distracting the mother or the medical staff
- The taper is ignoring more important responsibilities, like holding the mother's hand or otherwise helping her through contractions!

Is it rude to show friends photos or the videotape of the birth?

Let's just say you should be pretty *selective* about your screenings. I still cringe when I recall seeing, for the first time, the stack of snapshots my husband had been proudly showing neighbors and colleagues soon after our son's birth. While he had not photographed the birth itself, he had whipped out the camera just moments later, while our son was placed in my arms for the first time. And so there, amid close-ups of the little guy's face and the photos of our new family smiling together, were several shots of me holding the still-slimy Henry—with my legs still flopped apart. While they were beautiful shots, those few were also a bit, um, *bloody* for anyone but the nearest and dearest to have seen.

It's a good idea to edit snapshots shown to a wide audience. As for videotapes, use your discretion. If you ask first, most people will be too polite to refuse you, so be careful whom you ask. The majority of viewers may be made uncomfortable, as if they were invading one's privacy. Definitely don't show anything that the mother herself is uncomfortable with.

Birth is a breathtakingly beautiful event. Nevertheless, slight acquaintances, coworkers, and elderly relatives, in particular, might find offense in anything too graphic. Or the intimate nature of birth may embarrass them. The other party's comfort must come before the parents' own enthusiasm or their evangelical zeal for the wonder of birth. Children should never be shown such pictures without their parents' okay.

THANK-YOUS

How do I thank the doctor when it's over?
A verbal thanks is sufficient to a doctor or midwife. Later you can provide a photo of your joint success for the inevitable wall of babies in his or her office.

Too often overlooked is the equally important nursing staff, which typically spends more time with the laboring mother. My husband bought an especially helpful labor nurse a CD that we'd played during the birth that she had enjoyed. (He gave one to the doctor, too.) A small gift (a book, food) is so rarely seen by these hardworking women that they'll be bowled over. If your labor is long, the shift may switch, and you may be assisted by more than one nurse. Consider bringing a communal treat to the central nurses' station, such as a big box of doughnuts. Your partner can do this while you're still in the hospital, or you could drop off something later, with a note that recalls the birth: "Thanks again for helping me deliver Marcella Marie Smith, in room 222, the baby who took all day and all night on September 16 before she decided she was ready to be born."

SPREADING THE WORD

Is it the father's job to inform family members about the new baby?

Traditionally it was, since the mother was sequestered away to recover and the father was the one out and about. But in the age of cell phones and e-mail, not to mention plain old in-room telephones, that's no longer the case. Many couples agree in advance on a list of people to call. It's a good idea to write down all the names and numbers, and pack the list in your hospital bag before you go into labor. (Or you could pack your address book.)

When a woman has a C-section or a difficult birth, she might not feel well enough to make the obligatory calls. The father should inform the immediate family, or wait until the mother has rested. But if she's had a straightforward delivery, she is likely to be surging with adrenaline and just as eager as the new daddy to get on the horn and tell the world.

Is there a special order in which our families should be notified?

No traditions dictate this happy task, beyond common courtesy. If you have an older child, he or she deserves to hear the news first. Next tell the new mother's parents, followed by the new father's. Generally, everyone upon whom special status is conferred by the baby's birth—becoming a sibling, a grandparent, an aunt or an uncle—deserves to be high up on the list. If you're like most new parents, however, in your glee you'll be ready to tell anyone and everyone your headline.

Is it okay to telephone someone at 3 A.M. to deliver our happy news?
It's your call, so to speak. Bear in mind that while everyone is delighted to hear about a birth, not everyone appreciates such news in the wee hours. When my sister's son arrived at 1:38 A.M., she and her husband rang their folks and a few special others who had insisted on notification at any hour. Then she forced herself to rest. "I figured I'd get a much more enthused reception later in the morning," she said. (She did.)

CELEBRATIONS

Why is it customary to hand out cigars?
No one is sure how this ritual got started. It's now on the wane. Some people point to the obvious Freudian connection. Phallic-shaped cigars handed out by the proud papa remind recipients of his own role in the new baby. Farther back in time, smoke had a religious connotation, and setting a fire (or smoking a pipe) was a way to give thanks to the gods, up where the smoke would waft. Ceremonial smoking persists as a form of male bonding today—think men's clubs and smoking jackets—although in the 1990s, women began crashing those stereotypes as the fad for cigar smoking went coed. Handing out expensive cigars to celebrate birth may be an

extension of the ancient smoking ritual, combined with another tribal ritual, of a new father sharing his largesse with his clansmen.

Nonsmokers have plenty of alternative favors to share the spirit, including chocolates wrapped like cigars, pink or blue jelly beans, pink (or blue) pencils that say, "It's a girl (or boy)!" Some parents have special candy-bar wrappers printed up that announce "HERESHEIS." (Get it?)

Is the father supposed to give a certain gift to the new mother?

Custom calls for some special recognition of his partner's efforts and their shared new status as parents. At minimum, flowers brought to her bedside are called for. Some men splurge on jewelry, for example a pin or pendant featuring that month's birthstone. One father brought his wife a gold bangle for each of their five children's births, which added up to an impressive matched set.

More Ways to Celebrate Birth

Borrow a page from one of the many international twists on heralding a newborn's arrival:

- Fly a kite (Japan)
- Bring an odd number of fresh flowers—never even— to the parents (Russia)
- Toss colored confetti (Mexico)
- Surround the baby with foods he'll need to grow, such as salt, cereal, dates (Middle East)
- Play drums (Brazil)

- Plant a tree and name it for your child—apple tree for a girl, nut tree for a boy (Switzerland)
- Or plant a cedar tree for a boy or a pine tree for a girl; upon marriage, use the tree branches for the wedding *chuppah* (Israel)
- Open a bottle of rum (Jamaica)
- Serve red-dyed eggs—red symbolizes joy (China)
- Dress a newborn in clothing of the opposite sex to fool evil spirits (Great Britain)
- Sprinkle the baby with water to make him cry, which is said to protect him from later danger (Nigeria)
- Sing songs of joy (Morocco)
- Pass the baby around in a circle to family and friends, who whisper prayers in the baby's ear (Iran)
- On the twentieth day, take the baby to greet the sunrise (Hopi)
- Save the umbilical stump after it falls off and sew it into a cloth pouch that remains with the child through life as a good-luck amulet (Sioux)
- String red peppers outside your door to announce a son, straw to announce a daughter (Korea)
- String an olive branch outside your door to announce a son, woolen cloth to announce a daughter (Ancient Rome).

CIRCUMCISION

What if we choose not to circumcise our son but everyone keeps asking if we have?

The surgical removal of the foreskin around a boy's penis was once done as matter of course in the United States, just as surely as he was swaddled in a blue receiving blanket. In the seventies some 90 percent of American boys were circumcised. The tide has been changing rapidly, however. Today only about 60 percent are, and in some parts of the country the rate is as low as one-third. Circumcision is still the most commonly performed male surgery in this country, though.

Whereas Jewish men are ritually circumcised (*brit milah*) as a central tenet of their faith, as are Muslims because of the belief that the Prophet Muhammad was born without a foreskin, circumcision among Christians is a rather recent phenomenon. The practice only grew popular in the United States a result of the Victorian-era zeal for hygiene and a mistaken belief that it would curb masturbation.

Today, the medical community finds no particular health advantages to the practice. It is not true that the uncircumcised penis is more vulnerable to infection or penile cancer. To the contrary, the foreskin is believed to be a protective fold of skin. The notion that a boy will be better psychologically adjusted if he "looks like Dad" has also been discounted. As a result of this turn of medical opinion, increasing numbers of parents are questioning the need for the surgery. In 1999, the American Academy of Pediatrics (AAP) declared that the surgery is "not essential to the child's well-being." In recommending against the procedure being done routinely, the AAP abandoned its once-neutral stance on the subject. Worldwide, 80 percent of boys are left uncircumcised.

Because of the religious and social considerations involved, however, circumcision remains a personal choice for parents.

The sea change in its universality has caused circumcision to become a social question. "Did you have him circumcised?" is asked as freely as "How much did he weigh?" One's parents, grandparents, relatives, and friends may inquire about it. The trouble with giving a direct answer—aside from the fact that your son's private parts are, well, private—is that persistent questioners may then feel free to wander into even less comfortable terrain. Next they'll be asking whether the father is circumcised or not, or volunteering their personal experience with the subject.

It's your call, but you're well within your rights to nip the conversation in the bud, so to speak, by simply saying, "I appreciate your interest, but I'd rather not discuss it."

Circumcision: Yes or No?

The decision to circumcise a son reflects a religious, cultural, or personal preference. Some considerations:

Reasons in favor of circumcision:

- Your faith requires it.
- It is customary in your family.
- You feel that painkillers can numb the baby's pain or agree with those who believe the baby experiences little pain.

Reasons against circumcision:

- You want to spare your child unnecessary pain.
- You don't wish to expose your child to the risks associated with any surgery.
- There is no medical advantage to circumcision.

Can we invite family to the circumcision in the hospital?
Unless you are arranging a Jewish *bris*, circumcisions are con-

sidered a medical event, rather than a social one. There is no precedent or need for turning this quick surgery into a party.

HOSPITAL STAYS

Should one visit a new mom in the hospital without being expressly invited?
Hospital stays are so brief these days that it's best for well-wishers to wait until mother and baby are settled in at home before one visits. The exceptions, of course, are close family and friends whom the parents expect to descend upon them in the hospital. You can also ask the parents, when informed of the birth, if they'd mind a visit.

Bedside social calls should be brief—even if you're the new grandma—and done at reasonable midday hours. (Even then, the exhausted mom may be napping, and if so, should not be awakened.) If the parents would prefer that no one visit them in the hospital, they should notify the staff. Many hospitals will honor such requests and turn visitors away.

Is it rude to press for more time if I want to stay in the hospital longer than my doctor recommends or my insurance company allows?
Asking to bend a rule in your best medical interest is not an offensive act, so no offense can be taken. Tell your concerns to your doctor, or if your concern regards your newborn, tell your pediatrician as well. Don't be afraid to be persistent and to seek a second opinion if necessary. If the doctors agree there is just medical cause to extend a stay (for something other than mere fatigue), they may intervene with the insurance company on your behalf. It's also your prerogative to stay on at the hospital and pick up the tab. Or you could go

home and arrange for follow-up care from home-health aides. Most hospitals will help schedule this.

PROBLEMS AT BIRTH

Not all babies are born perfect. How do we tell people if something is wrong?
Either the parents or their family and friends can spread the word about the baby's condition along with word of his or her arrival. Divulge as much as you are comfortable saying. If the defect is a minor one and makes no difference to you, you certainly are under no obligation to disclose it.

Some parents find it helps heal their initial shock to discuss the situation candidly. Friends may be able to point them to resources for assistance, or to other parents with children who have a similar condition.

How does one offer help following a problematic birth without appearing pushy?
Sometimes the new parent of a child with a problem are in too much shock or denial to be able to receive friends. This self-protective response can preclude their getting all the help they can. If you are in the medical field or know someone who is in a position to provide needed assistance, you don't have to sit around helplessly. If you're not comfortable talking directly to the parents, or if you've tried that and been rebuffed, write a note explaining how you think you can help. Sometimes it's easier for the parents to think straight when the information is on paper. Offer in your note to follow up with a phone call in a few days, and do so.

What do friends and relatives do when they've heard that something is wrong with a baby, but not directly from the parents?

Once the baby is out of grave danger, it's appropriate to send a "welcome baby" card or gift just as you would if the child were born perfectly healthy. Just because a child is born with Down's syndrome, a cleft palate, or other birth defect is not cause to cancel the traditional congratulatory rites. A birth of any child is miraculous.

After the family is settled at home, it's fine to call to inquire how everyone is doing and arrange a visit. Indeed, sometimes friends avoid a family following a less-than-perfect birth because they don't know what to say or do. This only serves to isolate the family more. Your support and love will be very welcome.

Should well-wishers visit a preemie in the hospital?

Take your cues from the parents. Initially, the baby may be in too fragile a state. Many neonatal intensive-care units discourage visitors under certain circumstances. If the baby is to be hospitalized for several weeks or more, though, it may benefit from being stroked or touched in the isolette. Offer your assistance in this effort to the parents, though realize that they are probably content to handle this responsibility themselves. Don't be shy about asking the parents how you can help or whether the baby may be viewed.

9

Birth Announcements

"*It's a boy!*"
   "*It's a girl!*"
   The happiest days really are the days that babies come: Telling the world that your baby is finally here is one of the peaks of brand-new parenthood. The recipients of your glad tidings will share that joy. Hearing about the arrival of a newborn is exciting even when one already knows the baby's sex, name, and (sometimes) date of birth well in advance!

   Here's how to introduce your child with style and joy.

THE BASICS

Are formal birth announcements obsolete?

In our cell-phone, flash-mail world, few people receive word of a birth by the U.S. post anymore. Does it follow, then, that paper birth announcements are an anachronism not worth the bother? Not at all!

True, selecting the right paper and the right wording, and addressing and stamping all those envelopes, represent still more details to think about while you're pregnant (if you do this ahead of time, which I highly recommend). But these tasks can be a fun way to plan for your baby-to-be, just as decorating the nursery or buying the layette are. They don't have to be expensive.

A birth is a momentous occasion. Your child deserves a formal introduction to the world. And years from now, your child will appreciate seeing his birth announcement preserved for posterity in his baby book.

Who receives an announcement?

Send a birth announcement to anyone you think might like to know about your baby. That list might include immediate family, relatives near and far, friends, coworkers (including both spouses' immediate supervisors), and neighbors. It's also considerate to send one to every guest at your baby shower(s).

Ask your parents if they have special friends to whom they would also like you to mail one. (It should come from you, the parents, not them, the grandparents.)

It's fine to send a formal announcement even if the news has been preceded by a phone call.

Shouldn't we limit the number of announcements sent out because it's a veiled way to ask for a gift?

No. Some new parents are reluctant to mail many announcements because they confuse this piece of correspondence with a nudge for a gift. It's no such thing. Whether electronic, telephoned, engraved, handwritten, or silk-screened on a T-shirt, a birth announcement is simply a way to share your ecstasy—nothing less, nothing more.

You can leave your return address off the envelope, if you like, to subtly underscore that the announcement is nothing more than a way of sharing your glad tidings. It's correct, however, for recipients to acknowledge the announcement with a congratulatory note or to phone. But they are not obligated to send a gift.

TIMING

When are announcements sent?

Birth (or adoption) announcements should be mailed within four to six weeks of the child's arrival. Any tardier than that and even the most distant well-wishers will likely have heard about the baby, making even the formal purpose of an announcement seem a bit beside the point.

Some stationery shops print on site, which is one of the quickest and easiest routes. For example, I picked each of my children's cards late in my pregnancies, and then, on the day they were born, called the shop with the newborn's name and vitals. The cards were ready for pickup the next day. I had been given the envelopes to address when I first selected the announcements, so I also got that task out of the way before new motherhood hit. Formal engraved cards can take from six to eight weeks, so don't delay on placing your order.

TYPES OF ANNOUNCEMENTS

Which format is most proper?

Perhaps the most traditional style of birth announcements is a cream or white card on which the baby's full name and birth date are printed or engraved in black. This small card is affixed, with a tiny satin ribbon (usually pink, blue, or white), to a larger card printed with the parents' names. This format harkens back to the days of calling cards. Parents presumably already had their own cards to which the infant's card was attached. (With twins or multiples, each child gets his or her own separate card.)

Ribbon cards are undeniably charming, but have been losing ground in recent decades, not least because few of us use calling cards anymore. Some stationers require the parents to tie all those little ribbons on themselves—a time-consuming process that is worth inquiring about, should you decide to go this route. Traditional engraved cards are also expensive. (New printing methods can virtually duplicate their effect for a fraction of the cost, though.)

Formal ribbon cards have never been the sole proper way to announce a birth, however. In upper-crust circles, the preferred way was to write a separate note on good stationery to each person whom you wished to tell—and this is still a perfectly acceptable form today.

Fortunately for most new parents, there's a whole cabbage patch full of quicker and equally acceptable options for trumpeting a baby's arrival. You can have decorative announcements printed, use commercial fill-in-the-blank cards, make them on your computer, or come up with your own creative alternative. All formats are equally correct.

Some parents include a photograph of the newborn, which is a welcome touch. Even those who have heard about the birth before they received the mailed announcement will be happy to get a glimpse of the little one. Many hospitals use portrait services, which take the baby's picture on the first or second day of life. Alternatively, you could take snapshots yourselves, have them developed quickly, and order multiple reprints fairly inexpensively. Other photo options include digital pictures printed off a PC, or snapshots that are color-copied at a copy shop.

Where do I find birth announcements?

No one today can say that they can't find a good birth announcement. Sources of both ready-made and print-to-order announcements include: fine stationers' shops; card shops (such as Hallmark); department stores (look in stationery or baby departments); discount stores (such as Target); print shops (either local printers or chains such as Kinko's); party-supply stores; advertisements in parenting magazines (good for unique ideas); or the web. Check catalogs for samples before you buy.

You can also purchase special software and paper to help you create your own announcements on your computer.

On-Line Birth Announcements

Surf the Internet for ways to herald your baby's arrival to the whole World Wide Web. Examples:

- *www.my-kids.com*. Offers custom web pages for new-borns and families.
- *www.e-stork.com*. Posts photos, audio clips and video clips on private Web sites within days.
- *www.webnursery.com*. From First Foto; links to por-traits taken at participating hospitals.

Do e-mail birth announcements count?
As a means of spreading news quickly to a great number of people, electronic mail is even better than a cell phone in the delivery room. My husband sent off a quick bulletin about our third child right from his laptop within the hour of her birth. Bonus: you can scan in photos of the newborn, too.

But don't rely on electronic messages as your only way of introducing your newborn to the world. As an official an-nouncement of glad tidings, they're neither appropriately gra-cious nor very handsome when posted in a baby book for posterity. Anyway, even at the dawn of the twenty-first century, not all interested observers may be able to download fancy graphics. And you're bound to have a Great-aunt Helen or Cousin Pete who are yet to be wired. It's nice to order traditional announcements along with sending the news via e-mail. Or print your electronic message, with attractive graphics on good paper, to send to traditionalists and computer hold-outs.

EXAMPLES

What's the correct wording of an announcement?
There's no single preferred phrasing. At a minimum, of course, the facts to be included are the baby's full name, his or her birth date, and the parents' names. (You can either opt for formal names, Mr. and Mrs. John Formal, or the more familiar Mary and Bill Familiar, with the wife's name first, which has a warmer ring.) Nice optionals include:

- the day of the week
- the baby's birth weight
- the baby's length
- the place of birth (hospital and/or city and state)
- your full address
- any siblings' names
- the baby's Hebrew name (if Jewish; use Hebrew or Western spelling) and lunar Jewish birthdate

Some spoilsports say that length and weight data are irrelevant and should not be included on a birth announcement. But people are bound to ask for this ever-so-traditional trivia, so why not? (Do draw the line at giving details about Apgar scores or the names of your coaches.)

Aside from the basics, less is generally more on a birth announcement. If the announcements are folded rather than a flat card, you might include a relevant quotation from the Bible or other meaningful source on the front cover. Or on the front simply say, "It's a boy!" or "It's a girl!" (Or, "It's a boy—and a girl") Some announcements feature type-only, others are embellished by borders or drawings.

Whatever type of announcement you choose, under no circumstances should there be any references to gifts, or to where the new mother and baby are registered for gifts. Nor can specially printed cards from retailers listing this information be included in the envelope.

Here are some sample announcement wordings:

GENERAL

There is no single acceptable standard to follow, though the following wordings are traditional. (In place of "are proud to announce," you can say "joyfully announce," "are delighted to announce," or any similar sentiment.)

Augustine and Kenneth Newparents
are proud to announce
the birth of their son
Jacob Matthew Newparents
Saturday, December 23, 2000, at 8:20 A.M.
eight pounds, six ounces   21 inches long
Missoula, Montana

With great joy we welcome our beautiful daughter
Michele Frances
August 21, 2000
7 pounds, 11 ounces   21 inches
Mr. and Mrs. Bradley Hadababy

Louisa June Firstborn
June 24, 2000
Mr. and Mrs. Joseph Firstborn
Cincinnati, Ohio

PARENTS WITH DIFFERENT LAST NAMES
Whether you are married or not, your friends and family will
all want to know what the baby's last name is.

Jane Name and John Different
announce with joy
the birth of their son
Adam John Name Different
[Etc.]

TWINS
You can choose among different ways of announcing the
births of twins or multiples. If using ribbon cards, each child's
name is printed on his or her own card with a separate ribbon.

Mr. and Mrs. Frederick Duplicate
proudly announce the births of their twins
Paulina Ida and Colin Frederick
(six pounds, one ounce) (five pounds, three ounces)
Monday, November 27, 2000

If even one of the baby's names is used by both genders, you
might prefer to specify the gender

Karen and Tom Double
proudly announce the births of their twin son and daughter
Shelby Lee   Taylor Lynn

SINGLE MOTHERS

Don't shy away from sending birth announcements because you fear making yourself a target of frowns from disapproving relations. A birth is something to celebrate without regard to the circumstances. Do specify the baby's last name.

Tabitha Mary Singleton
is happy to announce the birth of
Stephen William Singleton
November 1, 2000

PARENTS WITH OLDER CHILDREN

Traditionally, a birth announcement contains only the parents' names. This is because the announcement comes from the parents, never from a child. (That's why the announcement ought not read, "Billy Bob is proud to announce the birth of his new baby sister.") But many parents today like to include older siblings, to make the older child(ren) feel special and in a general spirit of family unity. The trick is to not go overboard in playing up the older sibling. After all, the new baby should be the one who gets the emphasis.

This is the announcement my husband and I used. We deliberately chose the word "thrilled" because even more than "proud" or "happy," it's exactly how we felt;

Paula and George Spencer
are thrilled to announce
the birth of Henry, Eleanor, and Margaret's sister
Page Jubilee Spencer
Wednesday, August 18, 1999, at 4:01 A.M.
6 pounds, 15 ounces   19 ¼ inches
Knoxville, Tennessee

Alternative:

> *Winston and Graham Newsiblings*
> *have a new sister*
> *Lucy Louise Newsiblings*
> *born March 26, 2000*
> *7 pounds, 11 ounces   21 inches*
> *Brooklyn, New York*
> MARIAN AND ARTHUR NEWSIBLINGS

(list the parents' names at the bottom in a different typeface)

Or:

> *The Bigger Family joyfully introduces*
> *Our newest addition*
> *Bryson Robert*
> *Born October 30, 2000*
> *Charlotte, North Carolina*

SAME-SEX PARENTS

Use the same format as other couples would. Including the baby's surname will be helpful to friends who may wonder:

> *Sharon Female and Mary Ann Woman*
> *announce the birth of their daughter*
> *Suzette Female Woman*
> *[Etc.]*

WIDOW

A birth announcement is easily overlooked during such tragic circumstances, but it is proper to send one, if desired.

Mrs. Aaron Black
announces the birth of
Michael John Black
[Etc.]

PREEMIE

The wording of an announcement for a baby born prematurely is no different from any other. Because well-wishers may be concerned about a child who is born dangerously early, however, consider including a handwritten (or Xeroxed) "status report." Briefly explain what's going on with the baby, how well he's doing, and when you expect him home. To make the point of how tiny their son was, one family used hand-and foot-imprints to decorate their announcements.

OOPS!

What if you were expecting a boy, told everyone you were having a boy—but it was a girl? Follow the example of one clever couple who used card-style birth announcements. On the front were the words, "Boy Oh Boy!" And inside, "It's a girl!" with a picture and all the vital facts about their beautiful new daughter.

(For adoption announcements, see Chapter 11, "Adoption.")

Ways to Word It

There's no "right" way to phrase a birth announcement. Some ideas:

- "We're overjoyed to announce"
- "proudly introduce"

- "are elated to announce"
- "welcome with joy"
- "would like you to meet"
- "have the great pleasure of introducing"
- "Share our joy—it's a boy!"
- "We're in a whirl—it's a girl!"

UNUSUAL ANNOUNCEMENTS

Are handmade announcements passé?

Not at all. Some of the most treasured announcements are those that the proud parents have made themselves, assuming they have both the time and creative inclination for such a job. In addition to making a personal statement, you can save a lot of money by creating your own cards.

Some parents go for wordplay and puns. "Another step has been added to the Jacobs' ladder." Or, "The Katz Have a Kitten." Punny announcements peaked in the 1950s and 1960s. Traditionalists may frown on them, but the recipients usually smile.

Other new parents play off their professions. A photographer shot his wife in profile each month of pregnancy. He lined up all nine shots on a sheet of paper along with a tenth—his wife holding their new baby. A writer made her son's announcement to look like the write-up from the fictitious business journal *Young Executives in the News*, with the headline "B. J. Cole Hits Ground Running."

More ideas:

- Photograph your child wearing a custom-made onesie on which you've written the baby's name, birth date, and vital statistics in marker or fabric ink. Order multiple prints and mail them in fancy envelopes.

- Make photocopies of a wonderful baby photo and mount it on attractive heavy-stock paper. Use rubber stamps of ducks, toys, or other fitting motifs to decorate. You can also save time by having a rubber stamp made with the baby's name and birth date.
- Scan a photo into your computer (or use pictures taken with a digital camera) to incorporate the baby's picture right onto custom-designed announcements. You can get software specially created for designing unique birth announcements, including attractive typography.
- Use desktop-publishing software to create a newsletter about your new arrival. The first issue should highlight the birth. Subsequent issues can keep Grandma and other interested relatives up-to-date on future developments.
- Have a picture of your newborn made into postcards, with the vitals printed on the back. (Advantage: You only need less expensive postcard stamps, and no envelopes.)
- For twins or higher-order multiples, cut out a string of the corresponding number of paper dolls (the accordian kind that are joined together at the hands) and write a baby's name and vitals on each doll. Put the parents' names and the birth date on the reverse side.
- Cut out a miniature onesie from white flannel or a miniature-print fabric and glue it to the front of a plain card, with the baby's information printed below.
- Or decorate handmade cards with a rubber stamp made of the baby's handprint or footprint. To create this, bring an inked impression of the print to a rubber-stamp maker.

- Use ready-made photo cards (perhaps with a pink or blue border) into which you insert a photo and then write out or rubber-stamp the announcement. Such cards are available through catalogs or in retail shops.
- Draw your child's family tree. Sketch an actual tree if you're artistic or use calligraphy or nice typography to map the tree in the traditional linear way. Under your child's entry, include time of birth, birth weight, and so on.
- Use a ribbon to attach a hole-punched card or piece of paper onto "It's a Boy/Girl!" pencils. On the paper, write the child's name and birth date. This makes a cute way for siblings to share the news with classmates.

Can I combine a birth announcement with a Christmas card?

Provided your baby is born sometime after Thanksgiving, dual-purpose cards are certainly a time-saving alternative—and parents of holiday babies deserve all the stress-relieving breaks they can get. You could send Christmas cards in which you write a few words about the baby's arrival or better still, send cards that feature a holiday-esque photo of your baby (say, on Santa's knee or wearing a red costume). Or you could send traditional birth announcements and add a "Merry Christmas" note at the bottom. One family bought greeting cards with four stockings hung on the mantel, and wrote all their names—including the new baby's—on the stockings. News about her followed inside. If you had a spring or summer baby, it makes more sense to add baby news to a Christmas card than to add holiday greetings to a tardy formal birth announcement.

More Ways to Tell the World

Some exuberant expressions transcend common customs of etiquette. Feeling particularly flamboyant? You could always:

- Rent a billboard
- Plant a tree, with a commemorative plaque
- Hire a skywriter
- Launch some balloons or doves
- Wrap your house in a pink or blue bow
- Make your own wood "lawn stork"
- Design T-shirts with the baby's picture
- Buy a radio spot
- Have an announcement made at a sports game
- Take out a full-page newspaper ad

NEWSPAPER

Should an announcement be sent to the local paper?
This is the tradition is some communities. You can send your printed birth announcement or call in the information. Additional information that is sometimes included: the grandparents' names, the mother's maiden name (if it has changed), the hospital where the birth took place, the parents' occupations, the names of any older siblings. Some papers also print a photo of the baby. Check recent issues to figure out the preferred format. Some papers furnish a form requesting exactly what they need.

Sadly, this practice is on the decline because of security

reasons. Although certainly not an everyday occurrence, baby-napping does happen. The perpetrator is typically a woman who is desperate to have a child herself. Infant kidnappers target newborns, who they hope can be passed off as their own offspring. Often they scan newspaper birth announcements to find their targets. Granted, the risk is a small one. But it's for this reason that security experts advise against printing one's address in a newspaper birth announcement. Some papers merely note the hospital of birth and the parents' and babies' names, not even the birth date, and run the listings several weeks after the actual event.

10

Birth Ceremonies

*A*lmost every culture observes certain rites of passage to initiate a child into the community. They mark the importance and solemnity of birth. They place a child on a particular path in life. They perpetuate the group. They underscore our joy.

This chapter explains the whys and wherefores of three of the most common ceremonies new parents experience in the U.S. today: baptism, brit milah (bris), and the formal naming.

BAPTISM/CHRISTENING

What's the difference between a baptism and a christening?
The terms are essentially interchangeable. In both cases, the infant is formally named and welcomed to God's family. "Baptism" literally means "to dip." Biblically, the tradition comes from John the Baptist dipping Jesus in the River Jordan. (Children of the British royal family are still baptized with water specially drawn for the occasion from the Jordan, a custom dating back to the Crusades.) Children being baptized are either fully immersed in baptismal waters or sprinkled with water from a baptismal font. The word "baptism" is used to refer to the actual sacrament of welcome and incorporation into the church. "Christening" tends to refer to the naming part of the Christian ceremony.

How does one arrange a christening?
Start by calling your church office. You can do this before the baby's arrival or when you inform the church of the baby's birth. There you can get details as to how and when to schedule the service. Most Catholic parishes, for example, require parents to attend a preparation class (or classes) on the sacrament of baptism. If you would like the child christened in a church other than the one to which you belong, you may need special permission from the pastor.

Can we have our child christened if we're not particularly religious?
Few churches will turn away a family seeking to have their child christened. You may need to become a member of the congregation first. For some new parents, a christening is an event that brings them back in touch with their religious heritage.

When should it be held?
The preferred timing for a christening varies by denomination and congregation. Catholics, for example, traditionally baptized infants within the first two to four weeks of life, traditionally on the second Sunday after birth. This has more recently been modified to the first two to four months of life, so that the mother is able to attend. Other Christians baptize infants any time within the first six months, often later. Some denominations do not believe in infant baptism, preferring to wait until the child is old enough to make the decision himself or herself.

The christening usually takes place during a regularly scheduled church service or directly following one. The church may also have a dedicated service for christenings, often in concert with other families.

Don't be embarrassed to call your church office to ask

what's customary. Even if you've watched dozens of baptisms in your own church, if you're not experienced with babies, it can be difficult to tell their ages!

Where does the christening take place?
Traditionally the ceremony is done in the church, either within a regular church service or separately. Some churches also permit house christenings, which tend to be similar in ritual but take place in the baby's home. A makeshift font is usually created from a silver or porcelain bowl atop a table.

What happens at a christening?
The order of events varies by denomination and by congregation. Generally there is a welcoming and a statement of the purpose of baptism; a recitation or explanation of the child's name; prayer; and a rote series of questions and responses that reflect one's vows of faith. There may be also be scriptural readings, a discussion of the role of godparents, and a short sermon.

The actual baptism can involve the full immersion of the infant in water, or the sprinkling of waters on the child's forehead. If the baptism takes place during a church service, the infant may be "presented" to the entire congregation for their prayers and care.

Who holds the baby during the service (usually the mother, the father, or the godmother) depends on the ceremony. Sometimes it is a combination of different people. Let your minister be your guide.

Whom should be invited, and how?
Invitations to a christening should be informal—a telephone call will suffice, or a handwritten note. Commercial invitations are also available and can be used if this is common in your family.

The size of the gathering depends on your own traditions. For some families, the affair is limited to immediate family, grandparents, and the godparents. But in other communities, a baptism is a major social event. Many friends and relatives are invited to a large party at the parents' home afterward. Guests invited to a baptism need not be of the same faith as the parents.

What does the baby wear?
Who can resist the picture of a cherub-faced baby—boy or girl—decked out in a long, flowing white gown trimmed with smocking, embroidery, or lace? Called a christening gown, this is the traditional dress for the occasion. The gown usually consists of several layers of fabric that lies over a petticoat or two. There may be a matching bonnet and receiving blanket as well.

And yes, despite words like "gown" and "bonnet," both boys and girls wear such a christening outfit. Wearing white for a christening is a tradition that dates back to the long white robes worn by early Christians upon baptism. White symbolizes spiritual purity.

Some families have an heirloom gown that is passed down generations and among family members. While you are pregnant, start asking about the whereabouts of your family's gown to give the current owner ample warning to get it to you in time. If you're inclined to splurge and perhaps start your own heirloom tradition, christening gowns are also sold in better children's shops. For a unique gown, enlist a talented seamstress. Consider remaking your bridal gown.

A formal gown is a nicety, but not a requirement. Any white clothing will suffice, or you can swaddle the baby in a pretty white blanket or shawl. It's not always essential that the clothing is white, but the symbolic purity of such gowns is far more attractive—and age-appropriate—on wee ones than are pint-sized tuxedoes or velvet party dresses. Ask your church. In the Roman Catholic church, for example, the rite calls for a white garment to be presented—either the christening outfit provided by the parents or a white garment provided by the parish.

Older children being baptized may also be dressed in white, or in some congregations they may just wear their "Sunday best."

Children being baptized by full immersion may wear something more casual; they are then changed into a christening outfit after the water rite.

How do I handle it if I want to break tradition and not have my child wear an heirloom gown?

If there is such a gown at your disposal, consider yourself lucky! It would be a pity not to use it, particularly given the solemn and traditional nature of the occasion.

What do the adults wear?

Parents, godparents, and guests wear usual church attire. Because this is a special occasion, it's customary to err on the side of being slightly better dressed than usual, rather than the opposite. Sometimes corsages are worn by the mother and godmother, a slightly outmoded touch that is nonetheless appropriately festive.

Does one pay the clergy?

Yes, in some fashion. Exactly how varies by church. (Call the church office to ask.) If there is a set fee, or if some amount of voluntary payment is customary, it should be given to the minister in a plain envelope following the ceremony.

In some churches, payment is indirect. Catholics do not charge, for example, since baptism is a sacrament. But in many parishes a "stole fee," or special offering, is given directly to the priest, which is then turned over to the church. You may also make a donation directly to the church.

Some parents choose to present a gift to the minister, such as a book, collectible, or other special token to thank him or her for sharing in the special day. He or she (and spouse) should also receive an invitation to any gathering that you host in connection with the christening. Do not be offended, however, if your minister is unable to attend, given potential conflicts from other church duties.

Should there be a party, and if so, what kind?

A celebration following a christening is appropriate, although not necessary. Not every new parent feels up to entertaining, especially if the christening takes place within the first month. It's nice, however, to have a small reception right after the ceremony, with cake and coffee or perhaps a brunch if you're feeling ambitious. A catered reception is great for Mom if the baby is young. In some communities a potluck supper is customary. Ideally the celebration should be in your home, so that you can put the baby to bed if necessary.

A white cake with lavish white icing is traditionally served at a christening. It is inscribed with the baby's name or initials. The cake decorations are usually all white or pastels. Another fitting idea is to serve white-iced petits fours (small iced cakes).

Must the baby be present throughout the party?

That would be too much to ask of a social novice. If the baby remains alert and awake for the duration of the party, congratulate yourselves. But when he or she gets cranky, everyone will have a happier time if the guest of honor is sleeping rather than squirming and squalling.

Do guests bring gifts to a christening party?
Only the godparents are obligated to give something. For everyone else, if a gift has already been bestowed for the baby's birth, it is not necessary to give another at the baptism. You may bring a small token (a rattle, baby shoes), if you like. In some families, it's customary to give money for the baby at a christening.

How does one choose godparents?
A social significance has lately been layered on the religious one, with parents choosing their closest friends and favorite people for the role. Ultimately, however, Christian godparents (also called sponsors) are elected to be the child's spiritual guides and advisers. In some denominations, they speak the baptismal vows for the child, who will repeat them himself when he is old enough to be confirmed in the church. Godparents also assist the parents more generally, by taking a special interest in the child and providing help in whatever ways they can as the child grows. Among some faiths, these people are also considered the child's potential guardians in the event the child is orphaned. Simply asking someone to be a godparent does not automatically make him or her a *legal* guardian in the event of your deaths, though. To do this, you must have a will.

Some denominations may have special requirements for godparents. Catholics, for example, must ask a confirmed Catholic age sixteen or older. If you would like someone to be a godparent who is not Catholic, they could be paired with a godparent who is Catholic and would be called a "baptismal witness," serving essentially the same function. The witness must be a baptized Christian.

Likewise, the Catholic Church does not permit its members to serve as godparents to non-Catholics. The church does allow them to be witnesses, however, which is the same thing. Episcopalians prefer that at least one of the godparents be of that faith. Most Christian faiths require that the god-parents be Christians. Ask your minister to explain the re-quirements for godparents in your faith.

When selecting godparents, think carefully about who would make a good moral role model for your child. A person who is of the same faith might be a natural choice, although this is not always necessary from the church's perspective. Although special friends are customarily given this honor, family members are also excellent choices because you'll want the godparents to be people with whom you remain in con-tact throughout the child's entire upbringing. Do not ask ca-sual acquaintances or important people in the community whom you don't know well to take on this honor.

Parents are rarely their own children's godparents.

What are godparents' obligations?
The godparents ought to be present at the christening. In some denominations, they have merely a symbolic role and little to do other than stand up with the family. In other ceremonies, they may hold the child and repeat the baptismal vows for the child.

Over the long term, the godparents typically help the par-ents with the child's spiritual upbringing. How literally they carry out this task depends on the individuals involved. Gen-erally the godparents spend time with the child whenever possible as kindly, upright role models. They usually provide birthday and Christmas gifts, perhaps spiritual items such as religious books and music. Godparents traditionally give the child his or her first Bible.

It is not their job to provide the christening gown for the baptism or to pay any fees for the service. The parents arrange this. Godparents should give a special gift at the time of the christening, ideally something lasting such as a Bible, a cross pendant, or a silver memento.

When and how is one asked to be a godparent?

Because you want this individual to be present at the christening, you need to ask them before the date is set so that their schedule can be accommodated. You may ask while you are pregnant. It's best to make such a request in person, if possible. Underscore the reasons why you have chosen this individual, since you are conferring a special honor on him or her.

How many godparents may I choose?

Ask your minister. Most denominations employ just one set of godparents, but there are exceptions. Some Protestant churches permit more. Catholics may have just one godparent instead of two if preferred.

Can one decline a request to serve as godparent?

Being asked to be a godparent is a very high honor. It would be extremely rude to turn the parents down unless there were a compelling reason. Examples: a serious illness, an impending move, or the prospective godparent declaring that he or she was an atheist or agnostic, and therefore a poor example in the eyes of the church to be a spiritual role model.

Should each child in a family have the same godparents, or different ones?

It's your choice. Usually selecting different godparents allows you to distribute the honor more widely among your acquaintances without unduly burdening any one person.

BRIS

What is a *bris*?

Bris (or *brit* in Yiddish) is the Hebrew word for covenant or pledge. "*Brit milah*" means "the covenant of circumcision," a ritual ceremony in which a newborn Jewish boy is circumcised on the eighth day after his birth, connecting him to his Jewish ancestors. He is also officially named on this day.

For practicing Jews, the *bris* is not optional. One of the most ancient practices of Judaism, it's believed to be a physical act of faith that connects one to the essence of one's faith. Its mandate comes from Genesis 17:10–11, describing God's commandment to Abraham: "Such shall be the covenant between Me and you and your offspring to follow which you shall keep: every male among you shall be circumcised. You shall circumcise the flesh of your foreskin, and that shall be the sign of the covenant between Me and you."

All movements in Judaism—Reform, Conservative, Orthodox, Reconstructionist—mandate circumcision for their males.

When is the *bris* scheduled?

Circumcision is to occur on the eighth day after birth. In counting the eight days, remember that the Jewish day begins at sundown. If your child was born on Tuesday morning, then, the *bris* would be held before sundown on the following Tuesday. If he was born on Tuesday evening, however, the *bris* date would be the following Wednesday.

It's traditional to conduct this ritual early in the day, but there is no fixed preferred time. Your own family traditions can be your guide.

Are there exceptions to holding the circumcision on the eighth day?

If a baby is born prematurely or is sick (such as having jaundice or a more serious ailment), the *bris* is postponed until he's in good health. Usually eight days are allowed to elapse after the pronouncement of good health before the circumcision takes place. Confer with your pediatrician and your rabbi.

What if the eighth day after birth (or recovery) happens to fall on the Sabbath or another holy day, such as Yom Kippur? The *bris* still takes place on that day because circumcision is considered to be such a vitally important biblical mandate.

Exceptions: A *bris* is not held on the Sabbath or a holy day if it is for a child who was born by Cesarean section or if it is the *bris* of a child who's eighth-day *bris* was delayed because of health problems.

What happens at a *bris*?

There is no single *bris* ceremony. Usually a *mohel*—a special person trained to perform both the circumcision and the accompanying prayers—officiates. *Mohelim* (plural of *mohel*) are not necessarily ordained rabbis. A rabbi may co-officiate, but this is not necessary. In ancient times, the father did the actual circumcising. Today that's become a symbolic responsibility: the father arranges for the *mohel* to be present and may hand the circumcision knife to him, but he very rarely actually performs the procedure (unless he is surgically qualified to do so).

A *bris* ceremony has several parts: The circumcision (*brit milah*), the naming (*kiddush*), and, usually, a feast (*seudat mitzvah*) afterward. (The italics are Yiddish terms.) The occasion may take place in a synagogue or in the home.

The baby, usually swaddled in a blanket, is brought into

the room by the *kvater and kvaterin*, the godparents, or sponsors. Everyone stands during the ceremony, except for the special individual designated as *sandek*, the person who holds the baby during the actual circumcision. This honored role is traditionally offered to a grandfather; sometimes a grandmother or the baby's father fills the role. A close friend or relative may also be the *sandek*. The only requirement is that the individual be Jewish. (In some Sephardic communities, the *sandek* buys the clothing and blankets worn by the baby on this day.)

The opening greeting is "*Baruch baba,*" or "Blessed is the One who comes." The baby may be held down on a table or on a restraining board. After an introduction and a blessing, the *mohel* removes the baby's foreskin. Guests are usually forewarned, in case they choose not to look. It's even okay to leave the room. The parents say another blessing, as do the guests. This takes just a few minutes.

The *kiddush* is a blessing with wine, which includes the naming of the child. The *mohel* takes a drink and also offers some to the baby. The naming prayer is lengthy and explains the covenant of circumcision, and may include other prayers of thanksgiving as chosen by the *mohel* and the parents. Next the parents explain why they have chosen the baby's name and may offer other prayers or readings. Guests may also offer blessings. Singing often concludes the ceremonies. Finally, a celebratory meal is served.

How do I find a *mohel* if we are not active members of a synagogue?

To find a *mohel*, ask your friends or family, or inquire at a synagogue. Some hospitals in areas with large Jewish populations have a staff *mohel*. This is traditionally the father's job.

You can contact a *mohel* during pregnancy (even if you don't know your baby's sex yet) or right after the birth. You should discuss his fee (typically a set rate) and your preferences for the ceremony. He may ask you what your Hebrew names are, as well as your baby's, and will further prepare you for the ceremony.

Is a hospital circumcision sufficient?
Not to be recognized as a new member of the Jewish community. Circumcision can be performed several ways: by an obstetrician in the hospital; by a trained *mohel* in the hospital, or by a *mohel* at home. Technically only the latter two instances are a proper *bris*, because the circumcision is being intentionally performed to admit the child to the Covenant of Israel with appropriate prayers spoken. Some Reform Jews use medical doctors who are also *mohelim* to perform circumcision. They may also permit a physician (preferably one who is Jewish) to perform the procedure if a rabbi is also present to recite the blessing.

A hospital *bris* is the exception, rather than the rule, because postnatal hospital stays are now so short. Most Jewish mothers are back home by the eighth day. If you are having a *bris* in the hospital, it will be necessary to inquire about how many guests may be present and whether or not you may serve refreshments afterward.

Do we have to have a big party?
While a festive meal typically follows the circumcision, your *seudat mitzvah* does not have to be a grand affair. The important aspect of the *bris* is the sacred ritual, not the party afterward. Since the ceremony typically occurs early in the day, a simple brunch or a buffet/tea are good ideas.

Because this is a time of great celebration, a *bris* is often like an open house—people know when it is going to take place and just drop by. However, because the mother is still recovering from the physical stresses of childbirth and neither parent may be sleeping well at night, some couples simply send word that the occasion will be limited to immediate family. Other parents choose to hold a very private *bris*, limited to the circumcision. They then schedule a separate naming ceremony several weeks later, with a large guest list.

Your own family traditions may dictate how the celebration flows. But under any circumstance, the mother should not be expected to play the accommodating hostess on the big day itself. She should not be expected to do any of the cooking, the fussing over guests, or the cleanup.

Can non-Jews participate in a *bris*?

Yes. It's not necessary to be Jewish to be a guest or even an honored participant at a *bris*, such as a godparent. Only the *sendak* is required to be a Jew.

Must we serve kosher food?

If you do not observe traditional dietary laws (*kashrut*), you might find it an inconvenience to arrange for special foods to be served at your *seudat mitzvah*. Many nonobservant Jews are confused as to the details about what's permissible and what's not. A kosher meal following your ceremony is generally a wise idea, however, and may be required if your *bris* and celebration take place in a synagogue. It's also the considerate thing to do. Your *mohel*, rabbi, and some guests may not be able to join in the meal if it is not kosher. To find a reliable kosher caterer or receive instructions on what's permissible to serve, ask your rabbi or members of the synagogue for recommendations.

On what basis should godparents be selected? What are their duties?

The godparents—also called sponsors—are historically assistants to the *sandek* during the circumcision. Today these honorary roles are limited to bringing the baby into the *bris*. Traditionally, the *kvaterin* takes the baby from the mother and hands him to the *kvater*, who passes him to his father, who gives him to the *sandek*. Jewish godparents have a strictly honorary role limited to the *bris*. Unlike most Christian faiths, these individuals have no other obligations to the child or to his religious upbringing.

Clearly, however, the *kvater* and *kvaterin* are important honors. These roles are usually reserved for close family members or friends.

How are invitations to a *brit milah* issued?

There's little time to print and mail formal invitations to a *bris*, so informal telephone calls are all that is expected. The participants can be as few as the parents, the baby, the *mohel*, and the *sandek*. More typically, immediate family and close friends expect to be present. Given the short notice for the occasion, one does not issue RSVPs or expect an exact head count of participants.

What do the participants wear?

The importance of the occasion dictates appropriate dress. While formal clothing is not necessary, everyone should wear Sabbath-worthy attire. Because the *bris* takes place a week after birth, most new mothers will not have shed post-baby weight and will probably feel most comfortable, and look most attractive, in a mid-pregnancy maternity dress.

Whether or not headcoverings are worn in the home depends on custom. Be sure to have several extras for guest use if you are wearing them in your home.

What the baby wears depends on the custom in your community. Sometimes white garments are preferred, or dressy baby clothes are worn. The baby may be swaddled in an heirloom blanket or shawl or a special blanket bought or made for this occasion. Or he may not be wrapped in any sort of blanket at all. The boy may wear a small skullcap.

Can any chair be used as the Chair of Elijah?

It's customary to leave an empty chair in the room (sometimes draped with a special cloth, an heirloom scarf or shawl, or a personal memento such as the top of your wedding *chuppah*). This seat is for the prophet Elijah, who is said to attend every *bris* to guard over the child. The Chair of Elijah (also called the Throne of Elijah) is placed next to the *sandek's* seat. Any chair will do.

Is it proper to print up a program for the event, with the names of the various participants?

Many couples find such a program to be a nice addition to commemorate this special day. It's an especially nice memento if you include full text of pertinent readings, special blessings, or stories that convey the meanings of the names you have chosen for your child. It can also be a useful explanatory guide if many guests are unfamiliar with Jewish traditions or have not attended many *brises*. If you use printed programs, save one as a keepsake for your child's baby book. (A one-or two-sided photocopied sheet is sufficient, though you can get more elaborate as your energy and budget allows.)

Programs are not always practical, though. There are many things to take care of in the first week of a baby's life, and preparing a printed guide to the *bris* need not be a high priority. Some people may object to the rustling of paper as guests follow along, as this can interrupt the solemnity. Older relatives may frown on this relatively new custom.

Programs are also popular for girls' naming ceremonies, when there is often a bit more time to prepare such a pamphlet.

Is the *mohel* paid?

Yes. Each *mohel* usually charges a set rate. You should inquire about this ahead of time. If the *mohel* is being asked to travel a great distance (for instance, if you've engaged a family friend or a *mohel* from another town), you should also offer to pay his expenses. Pay him on the day of the *bris*. It's best to discreetly hand him an envelope containing the fee.

Can we hold a *bris* even if we choose not to circumcise our son?

Although ritual circumcision is a four thousand-year-old tradition in the Jewish faith, a small number of liberal Jews in both the U.S. and Israel are beginning to question its necessity. According to a National Public Radio report on this fledgling trend, their concerns are those that many parents have regarding the surgery, putting their baby through unnecessary pain. They point to Jewish law that instructs that it is forbidden to cause pain to any living thing.

Whether circumcision is central to the Jewish covenant or merely one small part of a complex mix of rituals is a matter of intense debate. You may find support or outright derision should you decide to buck centuries of tradition. If you are considering going this route, research the controversy in Jewish publications or on-line outlets, and talk to other parents and to your rabbi. Obviously much depends upon your congregation.

Because it's not technically a *bris* if there is no surgery, some families who bypass circumcision hold a naming ceremony instead.

OTHER JEWISH CEREMONIES

Shalom Zachar

What is *shalom zachar?*
On the first Friday night following a son's birth, family and friends traditionally visit to pay their respects and congratulations. If the baby is born on Friday morning, the *shalom zachar* ("greeting the male") takes place that same evening. Prayers are said and a light meal is shared.

Nowadays many mothers and their babies are either still in the hospital or lying low at home. Not everyone can withstand such a sudden influx of visitors. The ritual can be limited to immediate family.

A similar event, a *shalom nekevah* ("greeting the female"), can be held for a daughter.

Pidyon Haben

What is *pidyon haben?*
Pidyon haben is a brief, ancient ceremony reserved for a son who is also the firstborn. It means "redemption of the firstborn son." On the thirtieth day after birth, the boy is dedicated to the service of God. This follows a tradition wherein the firstborns of Israel were supposed to be dedicated to God and performed religious services for priests. The child is ritually released from these obligations with the payment of five dollars in coins.

Is a *pidyon haben* celebrated for a couple's first live birth after a previous miscarriage?
The traditional rules for this ceremony are pretty cut-and-

dried. *Pidyon haben* is not celebrated unless this is the mother's first pregnancy and the child is a male. A previous birth, miscarriage, abortion, or stillbirth—whether the child was a boy or a girl—would negate the observance of *pidyon haben*. Nor is it held when the firstborn arrived via Cesarean section.

Exceptions abound. Some reform rabbis now perform such ceremonies for children who are born following a miscarriage or surgically by C-section. And some egalitarian-minded parents have begun to hold a ceremony for girls called *pidyon habat,* redemption of the firstborn daughter. This ceremony celebrates the fact that any firstborn child is an important rite of passage for the new parents. Whether these options are available depends on the progressiveness of your synagogue and your rabbi.

Ceremonies for Jewish Girls

Is there a ceremony comparable to a *bris* for Jewish girls?
Obviously girls are not circumcised. Traditionally, a daughter is named the first time her father attends synagogue after her birth. More recently, it has become the custom to welcome a daughter with a ceremony that has all the joy and importance that sons receive at a *bris*. There is no single ceremony. Rather, parents may choose among several different variations on a naming ceremony that welcomes a daughter to Judaism. The ceremony is most often called *brit bat* (covenant for a daughter), but may also variously be referred to as *simchat bat* (rejoicing for a daughter), *Shalom bat* (welcome to the daughter) *brit Sarah* (covenant of Sarah), *brit bat Tziyon* (covenant for the daughters of Zion), or by other names.

These ceremonies are a relatively recent phenomenon, spawned in the 1960s and '70s as a result of the existence of the state of Israel, growing recognition of Jewish culture, and the feminist movement. Owing to its newness, there is no one format for this celebration. Most parents craft them from bits and pieces of the *bris*, the *bat mitzvah* coming-of-age ceremony, and even the *seder* and other ritual thanksgivings.

What happens at a *brit bat*?

Typically the *brit bat* (or other such rituals) is a brief welcoming ceremony at which the daughter is also named. (Jewish boys are named at the *bris*.) It can take place in the home or in the synagogue. The girl is brought into the room wrapped in a *tallit* or special blanket. One innovative mother used her bridal veil. There are usually prayers of welcoming and thanksgiving; covenant prayers that recognize the girl's place with the people of Israel; and the naming, at which her names are announced and explained, with recognition of the ancestors for whom she has been named.

You may choose to include other symbolic rituals. For example, some parents light seven candles, which symbolize the seven days of creation. Others include the ritual washing of the baby's feet, a tradition rooted in Sarah washing Abraham's feet. A newer innovation is to symbolically dip the baby in a ritual bath (*mikva*). Many families also reserve a ceremonial Elijah's chair for the Prophet, as is done at a *bris*.

Unless the *brit bat* takes place in a synagogue, it is not necessary for a rabbi to be present. The ceremony may be held at home.

As with a *bris*, it is customary to have a *seudat mitzvah* meal afterward. This can be simple or elaborate.

When should a Jewish girl's naming take place?

If the ceremony takes place in a synagogue, the first opportunity is often on the first Sabbath service after birth. But a naming ceremony can be held at any time. Unlike a *bris*, there is no one preferred interval. Some parents base the date on a religious significance: eight days after birth (as with the *bris*); fourteen days after the birth (the day a mother's ritual phase of impurity is thought to end); or on the day of the first new moon after birth (called *Rosh Chodesh*, a traditional day of rest for women, also carrying the significance of newness).

Who is invited to a naming ceremony?
Anyone you like. A large crowd is customary, since (like a *bris*) this is an occasion of great celebration. Or (like a *bris*), you may prefer to keep the gathering intimate.

Can I send formal invitations if there is time?
This is possible, but not necessary. As with a *bris*, it's customary to invite friends and family by phone.

What role do godparents play?
Godparents' responsibilities are limited to the naming ceremony (unlike Christian godparents, who traditionally play a broader role). A *sandek* (sponsor) may hold the child during the naming ceremony. Relatives or close friends (including non-Jews) are chosen to be godparents. They could hold the baby during the ceremony, read from the Torah, light candles, or perform other rituals that are part of your ceremony.

NAMING CEREMONIES

What is a naming ceremony?
Baby-naming ceremonies (also called Naming Day) are an increasingly popular way for nonreligious parents to celebrate their child's birth. In addition to formally declaring the name, it's also an opportunity to introduce your child to friends and

family and to share your happiness with others. The event fills a void for parents who are not active in an organized faith but who wish to acknowledge the spirituality of their child's birth.

Or that describes the modern American naming ceremony, anyway. Such rites of passage have been a staple of many cultures worldwide for centuries.

In Africa, for example, the naming ceremony is traditionally a major rite of passage that gives thanks for the baby's birth and formally bestows a name. The spiritual ritual is very festive, capped by a large family party. The Yoruba of Nigeria have created special Yoruban music, lullabies, and poetry for a naming. Many Muslims hold an *aqiqa*, a naming and welcoming ceremony, by the time the baby is a week old, or on the seventh day of life. A boy may also be circumcised at this time. A sweet is given to the baby, such as a softened date, some applesauce, or a banana. (The food just touches the child's lips.) Following a call to prayer, whispered in the baby's ear by the father, the baby is passed from guest to guest so that they may also whisper prayers.

In India, a naming ceremony is called *namakarana*. It is usually held between the eleventh and fortieth day of life. There are several variations. In one, mother and child are ceremonially bathed. A priest invokes a blessing, then the father whispers four names into the baby's right ear. The four names are 1) astrological, based on the constellation the child is born under; 2) the name of the deity of the month; 3) the name of the family deity; and 4) the popular name the child is known by. The child is blessed by Brahmins who have been invited for the occasion, and then gifts are distributed to the Brahmins and other relatives present.

How should a naming ceremony proceed?
It's up to you. Modern naming ceremonies tend to borrow and blend traditions and elements from a broad range of cultures. Most parents script their own ceremony. Often the parents officiate, in the absence of a religious leader. There is sometimes a spiritual dimension, in the form of prayers or religious readings.

Among the elements you may choose to include:

- *An explanation of the name(s).* Share why you chose them, describe their meaning. Consider including the surname as well. Some families elect the family's eldest member to perform this honor.
- *Meaningful readings.* They may come from works of literature important to you, philosophical treatises, or poetry. Or find a passage that relates to the child's name.
- *Music.* Perhaps special friends are singers or instrumentalists, or use recorded music.
- *Prayers.* Consider cross-cultural sacred words.
- *Group blessing.* Pass the child among those gathered so that each may kiss him or whisper words of welcome.
- *Contact with the elements.* Some naming ceremonies anoint the child with water, a sort of baptismal nod, or water is symbolically poured onto the ground.
- *Presentation of symbolic gifts.* Ask guests to bring something that will help the child throughout life, or to offer a wish for the baby.

Who is invited?
Whomever you choose. Some naming ceremonies are kept intimate in scale, while others are an opportunity for a huge party.

When should the naming ceremony be held?

Because the purpose is to introduce the child to the world and assign his or her name, this ritual is best held within the first month or two of a baby's life. Most families plan the event for soon after the mother has recovered from childbirth. But it can also take place later. Some African-Americans wait until later in the first year, or until the first birthday; at that time, they bestow an African middle name on the child (who presumably has already been using another name since birth). It's your call.

Where should the naming ceremony take place?

Naming ceremonies are usually held in the home. Parks, gardens, or other inspirational settings are also popular. Just don't count on your neighborhood church. Few clergyman within traditional mainstream faiths are apt to consent to a naming ceremony in the church, for the simple reason that it is a nonreligious rite. If it matters enough to parents to have the ceremony in a holy place, why not join the congregation and go along with church's accepted rituals? *Exception:* Individual leaders within certain denominations or faiths that do not observe infant baptism, such as Unitarian, Quaker, or Buddhist, may be willing to officiate.

May we select godparents?

This custom has been appropriated from traditional ceremonies welcoming infants to their spiritual family. Certainly there's no law against naming special individuals as symbolic guardians to your child. It seems a bit presumptuous, however, to use the term *god*parent in a nonreligious rite, particularly given that the Christian godparent's role is to serve as a spiritual guide. The preferable term for such a person in a naming ceremony is *mentor*—someone your child can look to for advice and guidance throughout life.

Can I hold a naming ceremony along with a christening or a *bris*?

It would be redundant to hold both a christening or *bris* and a naming ceremony.

More Naming-Day Traditions

- In Africa, the Yoruba call the baby Ikoko Omon ("newborn baby") until the naming day.
- In Tibet, Buddhist priests give babies a secret name, worn in a pouch around the neck throughout the child's life.
- In Vietnam, the father sometimes names the sons and the mother names the daughters.
- In Japan, the baby's name is announced at a gathering of family and friends on the seventh day after birth.
- In Uganda, the baby's name is spoken as he or she is offered the mother's breast. If the baby refuses to eat, another name is proposed, and this is repeated until the child feeds.
- In Thailand, infants are sometimes not given names until they are older, in the hopes that their anonymity will help them escape the notice of evil powers.
- In Ghana, a baby is not named until the seventh day, to be sure that he will live.
- In many cultures, a sickly baby is sometimes given a name that sounds ugly in order to frighten away evil spirits and disease.
- In New Zealand, a Maori priest recites ancestral names until the baby cries. The name that preceded the cry becomes the child's name.
- In Turkey, names are often changed or added at each

important life event, such as birth, circumcision, the first day of school, and marriage.

- In Senegal and other African countries, the child's name is whispered into his or her ear three times.
- In New Guinea, the day the infant smiles at his or her father for the first time becomes the Naming Day.

11

Adoption

The arrival of a child in one's family is an unparalleled high point, whether he arrives by natural childbirth, the court system, an adoption agency, or the stork. The only reason for a separate chapter about adoption issues is that people seem to have so many questions about it.

TELLING OTHERS

At what point should you tell people you're attempting to adopt?
While it's natural and sometimes vital (as in providing references) to let friends and family know when you plan to adopt, there's little need to make a more public announcement until your child has arrived. It's akin to letting the world know that you're now officially "trying" to get pregnant. Both situations are private and should best remain so.

Exception: If you are attempting a private adoption, not through an agency, you may find it necessary to spread the word more widely to make necessary contacts.

How is an adoption announcement worded?
There's no single established wording. You'll want to let people know the day the child came into your lives. You may

also want to include his or her age or birth date. If the child is not a newborn, well-wishers will be curious, and this may also help guide their baby-gift selections. It is not necessary to include the child's origins or other details about the adoption, although you may do so if you prefer.

Some examples:

> *Mr. and Mrs. Jay Newfamily*
> *proudly welcome their son*
> *Christopher Jay Newfamily*
> *who safely arrived Saturday, December 2, 2000*
> *Born July 8, 2000 in Seoul*

> *Jo and Lawrence Happy*
> *joyfully announce the adoption of*
> *Ella Louise*
> *Age: 18 months*

How is the announcement worded if it is from a single parent?
With similar phrasing:

> *Maribeth Solo*
> *Invites you to share her joy upon the arrival of*
> *Willow Mu Lan Solo*

> *Adopted: September 5; Born: January 17*

MATERNITY LEAVE

How much leave should I take?
An adoptive parent is entitled to the same amount of leave as a biological one. The needs to adjust, to bond, and to get

organized as a new family are the same. Take as much time as you are entitled by your company, and make no apologies for it.

How do I handle people who don't think I should take any maternity leave because I'm adopting?

Don't be pressured by itchy bosses or resentful colleagues into taking an abbreviated leave or none at all because you are not recovering from the physical trials of childbirth. Simply say, "I'm sorry you feel that way, but I am about to become a mother, and allowing my child and me to make that wonderful transition is what maternity leave is all about."

Make the same preparations you would if you were pregnant, including giving your supervisors notice of the impending adoption and planning how your work will be handled in your absence. In fact, you may need to make extra contingency plans since the exact timing of your departure may be difficult to predict. Do your best not to leave others in the lurch.

The same applies to fathers taking paternity leave, if their companies allow it.

SHOWERS

Is a shower appropriate if the adopted child is not an infant?

Mothers of adopted children are just as entitled to showers as mothers who go through a pregnancy. Despite the common term "baby shower," the age of the child doesn't matter. It's still a lovely gesture to welcome the child. If the child is older or this is not the parents' first child, the occasion might be better called a welcoming party.

If the child is not an infant, friends could bring clothing, books, and toys suitable to the child's age. The age (or birth date) should be noted on the invitations to serve as a guide: "Please come to a shower to welcome Maya, who was born in September." Or, "You are cordially invited to a welcoming party for Sue and Tom's new son, Kenneth, who is 22 months old."

Should a shower be held before or after the child's arrival?
The adoption process can be long and fraught with delays. To hold a shower before the baby's arrival can be unintentionally painful to the prospective parents. The baby toys and gear may gather dust for additional months, their presence a constant reminder of the child's absence. (Not to mention the fact that it's impossible to give the right-size clothing.) Should the adoption fall through, the parents must then face the sorrowful task of returning the gifts. It's far better to wait until the baby can be present at the festivities.

GIFTS

Is a gift sent when a child is adopted, just as when a baby is born?
Why not? Any new parent knows that the arrival of a child into the family is exciting, momentous, and celebratory—however he or she got there.

What gifts are appropriate for an older baby or child?
Clothing and age-appropriate toys are always welcomed because the parents are not likely to have any, unless there are older children in the household. Many traditional welcome-baby gifts, such as savings bonds or a personalized keepsake box are also suitable. (See Chapter 14, "Great Gifts.")

NAMES

If the birth mother has chosen a name, is it wrong to change it?

Even in an open adoption where the parents and the birth mother develop a close relationship, she has no legal rights to name the baby once the adoption is finalized. The adoptive parents may choose whatever name they wish.

If the birth mother has her heart set on a particular name and you wish to maintain a good relationship, it's wise to discuss the issue together. Explain why you've chosen the name you have and hear her out about her choice. You may want to accommodate her wishes by incorporating her selection as a middle name, but you have no obligation to do so.

Is it in good taste to give a child who is adopted a family name?

Yes. Not only is bestowing the name of a grandfather or great-aunt in good taste, it is a warm and lovely way to welcome the child into the family. The child is bound to grow up with an added layer of security thanks to this gift.

Can a child adopted by Jewish parents be named for their relatives?

Yes. It is traditional to select one of the parents' relations for a child's name, whether he or she is their biological child or has joined the family by adoption. If the birthmother is a Gentile or if the birthmother is unknown (therefore it is presumed she is a Gentile), the child is Gentile until it is formally converted. Under Jewish law, the relationship between adoptive parents and their child is the same as between biological parents and their child.

CEREMONIES

Can an adopted child be christened?
An adopted child of any background is entitled to be baptized by any Christian faith. The ceremony is usually no different from any other child baptism.

Does an adopted Jewish boy have a *bris?*
Yes. Because he is to be raised by Jewish parents in the Jewish faith (whatever his origins), an adopted son is circumcised as soon as possible, if not on the eighth day after birth. Infants older than a month or two are usually circumcised in a hospital under general anesthesia. All the usual rituals and celebrations of the *bris* are observed.

RUDE COMMENTS

How do I respond to nosy comments about my child's appearance or cultural background?
Few of those who blurt out such comments are being intentionally rude. Thoughtless, yes. Typically such individuals are unfamiliar with adoption and the language of adoption. They don't realize that certain comments ("How brave of you to adopt!" "What a lucky child!") carry connotations that there is something unfortunate or abnormal about your family. You can use such comments to subtly educate the other person. For example, "No, it's Bill and I who are the lucky ones, to have such a good baby."

Try not to be defensive. Remain gracious, but firm. If queries seem overly nosy, ask "Why do you want to know that?" It's possible that questions about a child's origins are rooted in the other party's genuine interest in adoption for themselves. Disclose only as much information as you are comfortable sharing. If your child is of a different heritage, polite comments about the child's nationality are understandable. You should expect them. Say something like, "Yes, she was born in China." But you are not obligated to divulge further details.

What can we do when relatives persist in referring to "your adopted son"?
Be polite but firm: "He's our son, period." It can be especially annoying, when you have both biological and adoptive children, for relatives to draw this distinction. Let them know that it's hurtful for you and for your child, as he grows older.

Responding to Rudeness

Most questions are blurted out in thoughtless curiosity— not that that excuses them. Here's how adoptive parents can deflect off-base queries:

When They Say...	*You Can Say...*
"Is she yours?"	"Yes, she is."
"But you're not his natural mother, are you?"	"I am not his *biological* mother, but motherhood comes naturally to me."
"Are you the real mother?"	"I really am his mother." Or "I feel pretty real."
"Which one is your real child?"	"They're both mine— they're brother and sister."

What They Say...	*You Can Say...*
"Why did her real mother give her up?"	"That's not your concern, but we feel blessed that her birth mother made adoption plans for her."
"Where did she get that bright red hair?"	"She was born with it."
"How much did it cost?"	"Raising kids is expensive, isn't it?"
"Did you adopt because you couldn't have a child of your own?"	"He is our own, thank you."
"I bet you'll get pregnant now that you've adopted."	"If we are lucky enough to have another child as wonderful as this one, that's just icing on the cake.

WHEN SOMETHING GOES AWRY

What's the appropriate response upon learning that someone's adoption has fallen through?

If the adoption proceedings were quite far along (for example, a birth mother changed her mind after the delivery), the parents may go through a period of mourning. Offer your condolences as you might following a miscarriage: "I'm so sorry." "I know you must be devastated." Your comfort and support will be important to them.

12

Visitors and Well-Wishers

*E*verybody wants to see a new baby. Who can blame them? There's nothing quite like getting the first glimpse of a new life. Does she have Daddy's chin? Mommy's coloring? Gosh, can you believe he's really here? Sometimes visitors are just as eager to catch a glimpse of their friends in action as newly minted parental units. For their part, most new parents are only too eager and proud to show off the fruit of their loins.

After a birth, many of the usual customs regarding entertaining get thrown out with the baby's bathwater. New parents' lives will run far more smoothly when both they and their company understand the following new rules of order.

FIRST VISITS

Whose duty is it to initiate visits—the new parents' or friends'?

This is one occasion where guests need not wait for an invitation to drop by. The new parents have too much else on their plates to be calling friends and inviting them to see the baby. You can be sure they do want to show him or her off. That's why it's up to the well-wishers to call and ask when a good time to stop by might be. Always phone first.

How soon after a baby's arrival may one visit the new parents at home?

So long as guests observe the supreme rule of new-baby visits—*don't stay long*—there's really nothing wrong with dropping by during the first day or two after the mother and baby have been discharged from the hospital. Close relatives, friends, and immediate neighbors will be itching to catch a glimpse of the newcomer. It's always a good idea to phone ahead, since napping is a primary objective in the house (the mother's napping, that is).

Should guests ring the doorbell, or would that be too loud?

Ring or knock in the usual way. Unless the parents have posted a BABY SLEEPING sign on the door—which I've actually seen some parents do—you can rest assured that most newborns will doze through most anything. Wise parents acclimate their babies to a certain amount of household noise.

LENGTH OF STAY

How long should visitors stay?

A meet-and-greet with a new baby should last no more than five or ten minutes. Most parents are thrilled to show off their little one, but they're probably not in the mood for a lengthy social call.

After the visitor has clucked over the baby's size and skin tone, bestowed a gift, and inquired whether there's anything she can do to help, she should make noises about leaving: "Sorry to rush off, but I've got to run some errands now, and I'm sure you want to rest up. I'll call next week to see how you're doing." Don't believe the parents when they kindly insist on a guest staying longer. At least, not for the first couple of weeks. After that, if their invitations to prolong a stay seems genuine, of course it's all right to do so. (Maybe they just napped, maybe they have a lot of help, or maybe they're a little starved for adult conversation.)

New parents should never feel obliged to encourage company to linger, because they may.

PLAYING HOSTESS

Is the new mother supposed to wear street clothes when well-wishers visit in the early days?
A new mom is most definitely excused from anything resembling dressing up. To the contrary, her goal should be to fix firmly in visitors' minds that her body has just undergone the momentous task of giving birth and she can scarcely tell her days from her nights. Receiving visitors in the first couple of weeks while wearing a pretty bathrobe is just the thing to remind callers that she craves (and deserves) her rest.

What should the new parents do when people drop by?
It can be hard to squelch deeply ingrained habits: You have guests, you take their coats, you offer them something to drink. But a new mother is exempt from such social niceties. Nor should guests coming to view a new baby expect them.

Well-wishers shouldn't expect a new mother to assume any hostess duties during the first weeks. In fact, the first four to six weeks postpartum was traditionally known as the "lying-in period" to reflect the new mother's need for rest and pampering while recovering from childbirth.

The new dad might offer refreshments. But the savvy visitor won't see anything amiss if he skips this ritual.

Can parents ask guests to please wash their hands before touching the baby?

Here's an exception to the rule that it's impolite to be nosy about other's personal hygiene. It's always a good idea to wash hands before touching an infant. Doing so always makes nervous first-time parents feel better. Phrase it in a gentle way, and invoke doctor's orders if you must: "I can't wait for you to hold Paulina, but may I first ask you to wash your hands? The doctor felt it would be a good idea until she's a bit hardier."

CHILD VISITORS

What if visitors want to bring children, but the parents think this is unsafe?

First-time parents tend to worry more about this nonissue than do veterans. One woman was so phobic about germs that she banished all children from the nursery—not even her favorite nephews met their little cousin until she was several weeks old. Of course, by the time her daughter was two and had a sister of her own, all those good intentions had evaporated.

Provided they are healthy, small children pose no special threat to a newborn. At least not medically—it's their curious pokes at eyeballs and their rocking the bassinet that alert adults need to be most wary about. Of course, parents should not bring a child to see a newborn if the child is ill or is known to have been exposed to a virus (even a cold, which can be rough on a newborn). When children visit, they should wash their hands just like any other guest. Show the child a safe place to touch the baby, such as stroking a foot.

GIFTS

If I'm given a gift in person, do I open it right away or save it until later?
Unwrap away! Your well-wisher is probably anxious to see how you like the item. If the giver doesn't care, she should say so: "Here's a little something for the baby that you can open later." Or if someone just stops by the house to hand you the present and peek at the baby, but doesn't wish to disturb you by sitting down to visit, you should merely take the package and open it after his or her departure.

Is it appropriate to give outgrown baby clothes as a gift?
It's the thought that counts with any present, not the amount you spend. Delivering a batch of beautiful, clean, well-pressed hand-me-downs might be very well appreciated by a new mother.

Remember, though, if they are given as a gift, the assumption is that you don't want them back. If the baby clothes are merely a loan, they should be presented as such and not gift-wrapped. But they should still be pristine and clean, and ideally the "best" things you have, items that it would be a shame to leave unused in a drawer. The giver should leave the strained-peach-stained stuff at home.

THANK-YOUS

Are in-person thanks sufficient for the presents visitors bring, or am I supposed to follow up with a card?
Technically a gift received, and acknowledged, in person does

not require a written follow-up. (Showers are the notable exception, given the circumstances of the giving.)

But since the person took the trouble to go to a shop, select the gift, wrap it, and deliver it to you, it's always an appreciative touch if you do put pen to paper and scrawl a hasty, heartfelt note of thanks. Alternately, you could snap a photo of the baby wearing an outfit that was given or lying next to a stuffed animal he received, and give it to your benefactor later.

Gifts that are mailed, rather than presented in person, do require thank-you notes, and relatively promptly. Thanks should be delivered within a month, ideally sooner. This is an exception to the general exemption due to new mothers about keeping up with social niceties. Make the task easier by keeping handy a basket of necessities: notecards, address book, stamps, pen. Newborns sleep a lot, and writing a quick thank-you note is not too taxing.

Your message need not be any longer than: "Thank you for the beautiful hooded towels. I know Jonathon will get plenty of use from them. Thanks again for thinking of us. Love, Lucy."

Is it tacky to write a thank-you card in the baby's voice, and sign her name?

There are those who will roll their eyes and think you've really lost it when they read a note like, "Dear Auntie Sue, I love my new blankie and I'm sure it will become a fast favorite. Thank you so much. Love, Bitsy." I confess that I have been guilty of penning such notes myself, in a goofy surge of hormonally altered new mommy pride. Then again, there are also those who will find such a message endearing (particularly some brand-new aunties and grandmas).

Use your discretion when lapsing into baby speak. A thank-you note to your boss, for example, ought to come from you. People without children may miss the joke entirely. But overall, the mere fact that you are writing a thank-you note at all is far more germane than whose voice is used.

Can I rely on e-mail or faxes to dash off thank-you notes?
It's better than nothing, and everyone knows you're pressed for time. Given the effort that someone took in selecting, buying, and wrapping your baby's gift, however, a properly handwritten note on nice paper looks far more appreciative.

PHONE CALLS

I don't have to answer every call, do I?
No. You shouldn't resent the flurry of calls that follows a baby's birth—people want to hear how you and the child are doing. But neither do you have to talk to every caller. Let your answering machine, call answering system, or your mate take the messages. Return calls when you're ready.

What's the best way to cut a call short if I'm exhausted?
With honesty. Yawn, sigh, or hold the receiver up to your bawling bundle. Then say, "Sorry but I've got to go now. I'll talk to you again soon."

RECORDINGS

What do I do when I realize that guests have heard me say something embarrassing over the baby monitor?
Ah, the blessings and curses of new technologies! Many a new parent has left on the monitor that allows her (or him) to hear the baby from another room, accidentally enabling others to listen in when she goes to tend to the baby.

Your best bet is to act like nothing happened. It may be embarrassing to realize that your visiting boss has just overheard you goo-goo, gaa-gaa over Poopsie's piggy toes but (assuming Poopsie is your baby and not your mate) your guest will probably find it charming that you're so in love with your baby. On the other hand, if you're overheard saying something like "Gee, I wish they would go home already!" you're apt to return to a room that's already cleared out. If your guest is suddenly chilly to you or makes a pointed remark about the monitor, your only recourse is to apologize.

How do I ask a visitor who persists in taking flash pictures of the baby to stop?

Unless your photographer friend is shooting an entire roll, one shot after another, of your baby at close range, there's probably nothing to worry about. A few pictures taken with a flash won't hurt your baby's eyes, not even if they're close-ups. If you're annoyed by the popping flashes, say something like, "That's plenty of pictures for now. Would you like to hold the baby instead? I'll take one of the two of you." Then take one last shot from a distance and turn the camera off. Alternately, you could position the baby in a place where there is plenty of natural light, negating the need for a flash.

BIDDING FAREWELL

How can I encourage visitors to leave when I'm tired?

You mean, what can you do when yawning, nodding off, or a red-faced squall from your baby have failed to give persistent visitors the hint? Ideally, a second person should be on hand with a new mom (your partner, your mother, a doula) who can help regulate visitors. It's always easier for a third party to say, "My! Look at the time. I think Mommy and Baby need to take a nap already, but I hope you'll call again next week."

If you're alone, you've simply got to do the dirty work yourself. Be apologetic but firm, not that you have anything to be apologizing about. "I'm sorry, but I need to cut this visit short. It was so nice of you to come by, and I adore the baby cup. It's hard for me to get up. Would you mind seeing yourself out? We'll talk soon."

Rest is the supreme obligation for a new mother, superseding all social obligations.

What do we do when it's our own parents (or other overnight visitors) who have overstayed their welcome?
Usually it's not the visitor, but the length of the visit, that's the problem. You'll need to convey this to your guest(s). No matter which side of the family your company is from, both new parents should sit down together with them for an honest talk. Underscore that you're glad they came to see your new baby and you love them, then load on the "buts." "We're tickled that you came to see the new baby right away and love you for it, but we are getting used to new parenthood. We're happy to show her off but we feel everything's upside-down around here and would like to have some time to ourselves with the baby now. Maybe if the house were bigger, it wouldn't be so hard but it is. Maybe when she's a little older, it will be easier. We'll bring her to your house for the holidays, which are coming soon. . . ." And so on.

RUDE COMMENTS

What's the appropriate response to a comment like "Wow, he looks like E.T."?
A smile—either weak or broad, depending how much you

agree with the observation. The fact is, many newborns *do* look strange. The ruddy, wrinkled ones tend to get compared with the alien movie star; the bald ones look like Uncle Fester; and so on. The person who makes such a comparison is not intentionally insulting your baby. They're merely being a little . . . tactless.

If you disagree with the remark, gently steer the rude person in a different direction: "Well actually, we all think he looks like Uncle Ned."

The better initial comment for a visitor eyeing an odd-looking baby, of course, would be to focus innocuously on at least one of his or her merits. (Yes, all babies have them, and usually in amplitude.) "Look at those nice big eyes!" "She certainly has beautiful skin." "I think she looks like you. What does your mother say?"

13

Life with Baby

*T*he rituals and celebrations regarding pregnancy and infants can be confusing enough. Everyday life with your bundle of joy introduces its own set of questions and quandaries. That's only understandable—you've never traveled around with a baby in tow before.

The good news: It's all easier than you think. All those rude folks who didn't know what to make of your sumo wrestler's belly seem to melt once you've got the baby in your arms. It's not that they'll forgive you anything, but they will give you lots of latitude.

SOCIAL OBLIGATIONS

Is it all right to ignore purely social correspondence for a few months?
For the first month or two with a new baby, you will be forgiven almost any ordinary social lapse. The first weeks after having a baby are a rarified time like no other in your life. You're getting used to a whole new person, body, and sleep schedule. . . .

Here are a few of the things no one is apt to expect you to do:

- Send birthday cards
- Send anniversary cards
- Write a weekly letter to your mother
- Check your e-mails
- Answer that college fund-raising appeal
- Correspond with your pen pals
- Make donations to your favorite charity
- Fill out surveys you receive in the mail
- Send cards for Christmas, Halloween, or any other holiday
- Respond to nonurgent faxes
- RSVP to parties (although you really should make the effort for big affairs, such as weddings)

These are all social correspondence. Ignore business matters such as bills, IRS notices, bank statements, and insurance inquiries only at your own risk. Institutions are much less forgiving than good friends following the birth of a baby.

Many new parents understandably don't want or need to let their social correspondence pile up. The mail delivery may be a high point in a day of baby care. Or they may simply want to tell the world their news and the baby's progress, old pen pals included. It's your choice.

After a couple of months of silence, however, people will start to wonder about you.

Can I bring my baby to a party if he hasn't been specifically invited?

It depends on the hosts and the nature of the event. When infants are very small and sleep a great deal, few people mind (or even notice) their presence. At a casual event, a newborn can be tucked in a corner in an infant carrier, or even worn in a soft carrier at a cocktail party or open house. At a formal event, an infant of any age would be out of place.

If you plan to bring your baby to an event, always ask your host if she minds.

Whether or not it's a good idea to arrive *en famille* depends on you, too. If you fuss a great deal over the baby, make a great show of diapering and feeding, and can talk about little else, you might not be ready for partygoing with a tot in tow. Better, then, to hire a sitter or stay home.

BABY RECORDS

What's the purpose of a baby book, and do I have to use one?
New moms seem to be divided in two camps: those who eagerly record every milestone, great and small, and those who record their baby's height and weight after the first couple of doctor's visits, and then stuff the book in a drawer and forget all about it. How zealous you are reflects your general tilt toward recording details, not how good a mother you are.

A baby book is simply a traditional record of your child's first year. It's easiest to use one of the many preprinted books available; some also include photo-album pages. (Some books cover the first five years, or more.) Or you can use a blank scrapbook of your own creation. Among the details that can be recorded:

- descriptions of baby showers (include a copy of the invitation, the guest list, a record of gifts received)
- sonogram pictures
- newborn's footprints and/or handprints (be sure you bring the book to the hospital to do this)
- copy of birth certificate
- copy of birth announcement
- newspaper or church bulletin announcement of the birth

- first photo, other favorite photographs (including a snap-shot of you pregnant)
- baby's hospital bracelet
- description of the birth and homecoming
- family tree
- record of baby gifts
- religious ceremonies (description, mementos)
- the baby's growth
- milestones (first time sat up, first solids, first steps)
- records of immunizations and illnesses
- dental chart (when teeth come in)
- first lock of hair
- funny sayings
- record of favorite toys and activities as baby grows
- annual "letters" that you write to your child on his or her birthday
- descriptions of birthdays, holidays, and travels

Baby-Book Alternatives

If you're not the baby-book type, or if you want even more ways to record your baby's life, consider one of these wonderful ways to preserve memories of the first year(s):

- A photo album with detailed captions
- A keepsake box where you toss mementos (hospital bracelet, first lock of hair, first shoes, medical records, etc.)
- A calendar on which you jot observations and "firsts"
- A diary

- A web page for baby (or for your family) that is updated periodically
- A scrapbook (which can include any paper memorabilia, such as welcome-baby cards, hospital bracelets, copy of birth certificate snapshots, written doctor's instructions, wallpaper or fabric scraps from the nursery)
- A special videotape where you record a minute or two of film every few weeks to watch your baby grow
- A cassette tape of verbal observations and baby sounds
- Collages of your child's special things—clothing, toys, blankets, cups, foods—which you then frame or photograph for posterity

BABY PHOTOS

Can I show off baby pictures without being invited to do so first?

It would take a cold heart indeed to be offended by a new mother or father whipping out snapshots of a bouncing baby. There's nothing wrong with pulling a few selected pictures out of your diaper bag or wallet, and saying, "I'm just too proud—let me show you how much Adam Michael has grown!"

Most people really do like to look at babies. But you don't need to walk your friends or colleagues through a frame-by-frame description of an entire thirty-six-shot role. They're most interested in who he or she looks like, how he or she has grown, or perhaps a very amusing bathtub or bearskin-rug shot. Few onlookers other than doting grandparents or eager aunties are likely to find much more than that as interesting as you do, even if they claim they do.

When should I have the baby's formal portrait made?

At most hospitals, a photo service takes pictures of the baby on the first or second day of life. But it doesn't really count as the first studio portrait. Often, the recuperating mother doesn't even know this has taken place, or she hasn't thought ahead to outfit the baby in her portrait clothes of choice.

You can have a baby's photographic portrait made at any time. Traditionally, the first one is taken at one month or three months. Price and the sort of look you want should guide your choice of photographer. Options include a large-chain commercial studio (such as JCPenney, Olan Mills, or Wal-Mart), a private studio, or an independent photographer, who may work from a studio or shoot on location (such as in your home). Check out samples of the photographer's work, particularly of babies your own child's age.

Many commercial photo studios offer packages that allow you to have your baby's picture taken at regular intervals (such as at three months, six months, and twelve months) at a discount. Don't expect miracles of the one-month or three-month shoot, though. Young infants sometimes look squinched if they are propped up in a sitting position. It's better if the baby can hold her head up while positioned on her belly, or if photographed in your arms.

Perhaps the most wonderful age to photograph a baby is six months. I say this as a portrait-happy mother whose favorite pictures of each child was made at this age. A friend's mother had all seven of her children photographed at six months in black-and-white. The identically-framed faces line a long hallway in their home—a sight heartwarming enough to almost make you want to have seven kids yourself. (Almost.)

Why is six months such a camera-friendly age? By then, most babies can sit up well and grin broadly. Yet they're usually not able to crawl out of the frame yet. Nor has stranger anxiety (causing them to burst into tears at the sight of the photographer) kicked in. Best of all, they still have all that adorable plumpness. They look just the way babies are supposed to look.

Even if you or your partner are devoted amateur shutterbugs who constantly record your little one, a portrait by a pro is a worthy investment. Your cherub won't stay tiny for very long. There's something especially charming and eternal about a professionally lit image. And it's the perfect birthday or Christmas present for Grandma and Grandpa!

What should the baby wear in a portrait?
Your photographer of choice may make suggestions. In general, choose something with simple lines and a minimal pattern. You want the baby to pop out of the picture frame, not the clothes. White is a perfect color, although pastels also lend that cute-as-can-be look. Don't worry about buying special shoes for a prewalker; pretty socks or bare feet look natural. Skip the jewelry and heavy layers of lace and crinolines for girls, and leave home the mini-three-piece-suits for boys. Dress your baby to look like the innocent child he or she is. Or try a birthday suit.

OUTINGS

Can I take a newborn to a restaurant?
My third child dined out for the first time when she was three days old. Since my parents were in town, they made handy baby-sitters for Margaret's older siblings, and because she was still so young, she did nothing but sleep. We figured we might not have another opportunity as good as this for quite a while!

If the mother feels up to it, there's no reason not to bring a newborn to a restaurant. If you have a removable car seat that doubles as a carrier, your child may sleep right through the transition from car to building. The parents should never be goaded into going out, however. New moms may not yet feel comfortable handling and feeding a newborn and prefer to wait a few weeks before going out.

Can I bring my baby to the office during my maternity leave?

Your colleagues may be as eager as your friends and relatives to see your little one—once, or maybe twice. Should you drop by more often than that, your presence is apt to be a distraction, and you risk whipping up hidden resentments. Rightly or wrongly, people may think, *Well if she's got so much time to hang around here, why isn't she back on the job?*

Choose a day in the middle of your leave when you are feeling well. It's a good idea to prearrange the timing of your visit with a coworker to be sure you're not intruding on a big meeting or other important office event. Make the rounds briefly to show off your baby, and then leave. (Or go to lunch with a close friend or two from the office; you can visit as long as you like off the premises.) Don't overstay your welcome. You also risk getting wrangled into helping out "with just this one problem" or somesuch. Maternity leave means that you leave office matters behind for a set period, as well you should.

It is rude to bring strollers into stores—so many people seem to frown?

Certainly mothers with babies have as much right to be out and about as anyone—and are perhaps in more need of the exercise and mental stimulation than the average person. But use common sense when planning outings. Think about your destination and how crowded it's liable to be.

Parents must constantly balance their own need to make things as easy as possible against the convenience of others. Thus, a full-size stroller in a half-empty shopping mall at ten o'clock in the morning is fine. A full-size stroller in a snug shop the week before Christmas is a potential irritant to everyone. Carriages are handy for small babies who sleep a lot, but they can also be a hassle to fold and unfold and to navigate through crowds. Consider wearing your small baby in a sling when shopping. Umbrella strollers (once a baby can sit up, around six months) are easier to maneuver and take up less room than do large strollers. Stash one in the trunk of your car so it'll be there whenever you need it.

BREAST-FEEDING

Is it okay to breast-feed in public?
Absolutely. Don't let anyone make you feel embarrassed, guilty, or improper by nursing your baby whenever, and wherever, she's hungry.

I've opened my shirtfront in stores and restaurants, during parties and church services, in front of my dad and in front of my boss, and once, memorably, in the middle seat of an airplane between two suited businessmen who suddenly became very absorbed in their paperwork. The baby wants food, and I have it. Just as I'd offer a bag of goldfish crackers to a three-year-old, why would I hesitate to put a baby to my breast? Providing sustenance is part of a mother's job description.

Unfortunately the issue of public breast-feeding is not always so straightforward in America. While the vast majority of moms are able to do so without a word of criticism (and usually without anyone noticing), bizarre exceptions make the papers all the time. "It's bad for the children to see," a mother in a New Jersey toy store was told. "No food is allowed at the pool," was another line. And, "Sorry, but I don't allow people to have intercourse in here, either." My favorite is the mom attending an outdoor concert in Washington, DC, who was informed that breast-feeding would "attract bees." These excuses would be pretty funny, if they didn't affect real, needy infants and real, unnerved mothers.

Ironically, more is now known about the benefits of breast-feeding than when our grandmothers did so routinely, when it was considered a natural extension of pregnancy. Breast-feeding lowers the risk of SIDS, provides immunities against diseases ranging from ear infections to pneumonia, and has been linked to higher IQ. Women who breast-feed have lower rates of urinary-tract infections, osteoporosis, breast cancer, uterine cancer, and ovarian cancer. The American Academy of Pediatrics recommends breast milk for the first year of life.

Too often, though, women quit (or fail to start) because breast-feeding is virtually invisible in our culture, says Mary Lofton, a La Leche League International spokeswoman in Schaumburg, Illinois. In Europe and Australia, for example, public breast-feeding is the norm.

Some critics claim that because observers may be made uncomfortable by seeing a mother breast-feed, it follows that she shouldn't do it. But this is both out-of-date and illogical. Some people are made uncomfortable by watching others eat sushi. Besides, breast-feeding is not a private act akin to brushing one's hair or taking a shower. It's the feeding of another human being. Anyone who is uncomfortable to be in the presence of a nursing mother is focusing a little too much on the process. You're actually doing other mothers a favor by nursing in public—seeing your example may embolden them.

Is there anyplace one should not breast-feed?
Yes. A rest room. Unless there is a lounge attached with comfortable seating, a bathroom is the dirtiest, least pleasant, and least appropriate place to nurse.

What do I do if I sense that others don't approve of public breast-feeding?
The most important ingredient of successful breast-feeding wherever you need to is to feel comfortable yourself. Here's how:

- *Don't worry about everybody else.* Feeling overly self-conscious can inhibit milk let-down. Worse, you may wind up quitting sooner than is optimal for your baby's health. Remind yourself that the vast majority of people are supportive of a woman's need to nourish her child. It's what breasts were meant to do. Focus on the only person who ultimately needs to care about what you're doing: your baby.

- *Practice.* Rehearse in front of a full-length mirror. Bring your baby close to your body, unfasten your shirt and bra, and help her latch on. Rearrange your clothing or a blanket around your baby's face. Then look up as if you were continuing to talk to a friend or people-watch. By watching yourself, you'll be able to see how natural and unobtrusive breast-feeding really looks. (Most onlookers will think your baby is asleep, anyway.)

- *Dress for convenience.* One woman will never forget a meeting with a lawyer when her daughter was two weeks old. "I naively thought she'd sleep. I had on a button-down shirt. When she began to scream. I had no choice but to bare all," she said. "It was embarrassing even though the attorney was great. I learned the lesson of never going out without a nursing top on."

"I'll be the first to say that you don't need special clothes in order to breast-feed," insists Jody Wright, owner of Motherwear, a wonderful mail-order catalog of nursing clothes based in Northampton, Massachusetts. She knows about the value of discretion, though, having received her share of stares for breast-feeding her adopted children, who are of a different race. Some women favor strapless bras or stretchy athletic models under roomy T-shirts. Almost any front-opening top works fine, although many reveal more skin than do nursing designs, which feature different kinds of concealed openings that make public nursing less obvious. (Nursing dresses are especially convenient, since it can be hard to find a regular dress that's accessible.) At the beach, try a T-shirt over your swimsuit.

- *Dress for camouflage.* Since it's common for the opposite breast to leak during a feeding, absorb excess fluid with breast pads (made of cut-up old T-shirts or bought in reusable or disposable form from a store). Print fabrics hide stains more effectively than plain. Some manufacturers (including Motherwear) sell baby outfits in the same fabrics as the mother's clothes, so the two of you blend together.

- *Cover up.* For extra discretion, the easiest tactic is a receiving blanket (or scarf, shawl, or blazer) tossed over your shoulder. A brimmed hat on the baby also helps hide the nipple. Some women prefer the privacy of a cloth sling-style carrier.

- *Create your own privacy zone.* If you look at your clothes as you unfasten them or at your baby as he nurses, others will follow your gaze. Instead, meet people's eyes and smile, or create a private space with the positioning of your body. Turn slightly away to signal that you're not available for interactions, Jody Wright suggests, or focus on a book. At restaurants, choose a private booth or a table out of the traffic flow.

- *But don't go overboard in your zeal to be discreet.* "Some women try so hard—they turn their chairs backward, use a shawl, and wind up drawing more attention to themselves," says Elizabeth Baldwin, a legal adviser to La Leche League, the international breast-feeding support organization. "People in our society are often not so upset by the exposure of breast-feeding as the mere thought of it." With experience, you'll be able to nurse while carrying on normally.

- *Time your outings.* As you learn your baby's signals, you can pick out a comfortable spot to nurse at the first sign of hunger fussing, before whimpers turn to wails. Some moms nurse in their parked cars before heading into places like banks or groceries where it can be hard to sit. Older children may understand if you firmly say to wait until you get to a quiet place (so long as you follow through promptly); many mothers find that nursing a toddler in public is tricky because kids this age are so distractible.

- *Politely deflect criticism.* Dirty looks or rude words are rare, but upsetting. If they happen to you, hold your ground. Don't be intimidated into retreating into a dirty bathroom. Tell the critic that you're doing what's best for your baby, and that it's your baby's right to breast-feed anywhere. Point out that you're considering others' feelings by being discreet. By speaking up, you're helping educate the ignorant, and by staying put, you're an encouraging example to others.

- *Rest assured that it gets easier.* New moms are often the most ill at ease with public breast-feeding because everything about handling a newborn is unfamiliar.

What about pumping milk in front of others?
Because this is neither a natural nor familiar act, and the noise of a pump (or the motions of doing so by hand) attracts attention, it is extremely difficult to pump milk discreetly. Therefore, this everyday act, however necessary, must be considered one that the world at large is not quite ready to observe. A mother should retire to a private room to pump milk. It's all right to do so in front of a relative or a close friend, however, if you are sure they are not made uncomfortable.

Comebacks for Breast-feeding Snipes

Remind yourself that a lack of understanding about the importance of breast-feeding is generally behind strange, rude comments observers will come up with.

When They Say . . .	*You Can Say . . .*
"You should use the bathroom."	"Would you want to eat your lunch in there?"
"You wouldn't let your child urinate right out here, would you?"	"No, but I would let him eat here, which is what my baby is doing"
"No eating is allowed here."	"Don't worry. There won't be any crumbs and he won't share."
"That's not natural."	"It's more natural than bottle-feeding."

What They Say...	*You Can Say...*
"Breasts are sexual. They belong in the bedroom, not out in public."	"*Sometimes* breasts are sexual, but right now they're functional—they're feeding my baby."
"You're making other people uncomfortable."	"I think they'd be a lot more uncomfortable listening to my baby scream because he was hungry."
"How do you know if she's getting enough?"	"When she's had enough, she'll stop."

What do I say to people who criticize me for not breast-feeding?

While some enthusiasts would like to make a political issue out of breast-feeding, it is ultimately a personal choice. Ideally, women should keep an open mind, before the baby's birth, about whether or not to nurse. A small percentage of women have no choice in the matter, though. They are physically unable to breast-feed (because of some types of breast implants or breast reduction surgery, because of seriously inverted nipples, or because their bodies cannot manufacture sufficient milk, among other reasons).

Once the child has arrived, anyone who comments on the mother's feeding decision is out of line. Sure, breast is best, but today's infants thrive on high-tech, high-quality formula as well. Probing—or worse, criticizing—a mother for what's in her baby's bottle (which could be expressed breast milk, for all the intruder knows) is akin to accosting a fellow restaurant patron for buttering her roll or ordering steak instead of the vegetarian special. It's just not done.

To the question "Why aren't you breast-feeding?" a mother need only say, "I'm sorry, but that really isn't any of your business." Whether you launch into the details is your right, but not your obligation. Some women who cannot breast-feed find that offering an explanation helps assuage their own sense of guilt or inadequacy, although this approach can also leave the mother vulnerable to uninformed advice that only makes her feel worse. It helps if you can feel comfortable with your feeding choice quickly, breast or formula. Don't get roped into debates or guilt trips once your baby has arrived. You've got more pressing matters to think about, like whether he needs a new diaper yet and how much spit up has just slimed your shoulder.

DIAPERING

Where may I change a diaper in public?
The first, best place to go is to a rest room with baby-changing facilities. Typically these are a special counter or a pull-down shelf designated for diaper changing. They tend to be a comfortable height for the job and feature a safety belt to keep the baby in place (not that you should take your hand off of him for a second). These facilities are becoming commonplace everywhere from fast-food restaurants to shopping malls to bookstores. Nicest of all, they appear almost as often in men's rooms as in women's.

If a bathroom does not have changing facilities, however, it is probably the last place you should go to change your baby's diaper. With the exception of swanky bathrooms that have separate lounge rooms, a public bathroom tends to be cramped and filthy. You sure wouldn't want to lay the baby on the floor, not even with a changing mat from your diaper bag between his bottom and the infested floor.

So long as you're fast, hygienic, and discreet, you can safely change a young baby's diaper almost anywhere. Depending where you are, ask if there's a spare room or closet available. Failing that, choose a quiet corner out of the way. (Off-limits: at a restaurant within view of other diners, no matter how speedy you are.) Sometimes it's easiest to make a quick change in your car or outside, on a park bench. Carry a changing pad, diapers, and a supply of wet baby wipes in your diaper bag wherever you go.

DEPRESSION

How should one intervene if they sense a new mom is suffering from postpartum depression?
Both the placenta and the fetus produce hormones during pregnancy. When they are delivered, hormonal levels plummet. Probably as a result, about two to four days after delivery, up to eighty percent of new moms are surprised to find their feelings of joy tempered by moodiness, crying jags, and depression. These so-called "baby blues" usually fade within a week, almost as suddenly as they arrived.

For ten to twenty-five percent of new moms, a type of depression lingers. It can appear at any time during the baby's first year, generally within the first two months, and last for up to a year. Symptoms of postpartum depression (known as PPD) include trouble sleeping or eating, anxiety, lack of confidence, detachment, pessimism, and anger toward others or the baby. Often women fail to recognize a problem, because they think, "This must be what motherhood is like." Or they're aware something's wrong but feel too ashamed to tell anyone. In fact, PPD is a very real biological disorder.

If you suspect this is the case with someone you know, the first best thing you can do is to broach the subject. She may not be aware that PPD exists, or be familiar with its symptoms. Chances are good that she will be relieved to put a name to her distressing feelings, and to have someone to discuss them with. Encourage her to mention her symptoms to her doctor.

Also be sure that the woman is getting as much help with baby care as she can. A lack of social support can intensify the reaction. PPD is less common in cultures that have a lot of support rituals for new moms, including emotional and practical support. Rest and just talking to others can ease mild cases. It especially helps to compare notes with other new moms about what's normal. Suggest a mothers' group, postpartum exercise class, or on-line chat group.

BABY-SITTERS

Is it forward to volunteer to baby-sit?
Offering well-meant assistance is never too forward, especially where it concerns helping out with a new baby. If the parents aren't comfortable leaving their child yet, they need only thank you and politely decline. Offer a raincheck for when the baby is a bit older. They're apt to be eternally grateful.

Can I take up friends on offers they have made in the past to baby-sit?
No one should make an offer that they aren't fully prepared to live up to. So if someone has volunteered to baby-sit for you, whether the offer was made during your pregnancy or after, you most certainly may call him or her on it. Many veteran parents welcome the chance to be around a small baby once again, and prospective parents may be eager to sample the experience.

Most people are happy to help out, especially when babies are young and not too mobile or demanding.

Should relatives who baby-sit be paid?

Although they may decline money because they are baby-sitting out of genuine love and a desire to help out, relatives who baby-sit can correctly be offered it. If you are sure they might take offense, instead say something like, "Oh it's so nice of you to do this. However can we thank you?" Even if your kind mother or sister says, "It's my pleasure; don't worry about it," you can look for ways to repay the kindness later. Send flowers, pick up a trinket for her on vacation, fix her lawn-mower, and so forth.

If a relative baby-sits for you on a regular basis, such as providing child care while you work, it's best to work out a fair payment plan in advance.

How do I let a friend know that I think the sitter she's recommended is not right for me?

Well-meaning friends are often happy to share baby-sitter contacts with new friends. But a friend's recommendation alone is not reason enough to hire a sitter. You absolutely must be comfortable with the person yourselves.

Parents of young babies are often most comfortable with mature baby-sitters. Not only do older people have experience caring for infants, their maturity is soothing when you're unaccustomed to leaving your child. Preteens, even conscientious ones, can be too careless to entrust with a newborn. Many parents draw the line at anyone younger than eighteen.

Be frank with your friend without criticizing her judgement. "Thanks for suggesting Mary Lou. I'm sure she's great with your child, but we are really more comfortable with someone older." Or, "I appreciate your giving me Darla's phone number, but I think we'll just stick to relatives as baby-

sitters until we get a little more experienced at parenthood."
She should not take your rejection of the suggestion as an
implication that she's employing an inferior baby-sitter herself. Nor should you intimate that.

What's the going rate for baby-sitting?

Rates vary by community. They may also be influenced by
such factors as the age of the child, the age of the sitter, the
number of children, and whether it's an occasional or regular
job. You'll want to pay a fair market rate if you want to retain
a good sitter. Resist the temptation to underpay. Even if your
baby will merely be sleeping during most of the evening,
you're paying for the security of knowing your most priceless
possession is in good hands.

To find out what the rates are in your area, ask other parents of children the same age as yours. Also ask your sitter
what her customary rates are. When more than one child is
being watched, rates should be incrementally higher.

Agree upon the rate (usually hourly) before the sitter arrives. Pay the sitter at the end of the evening, ideally in cash.

Tips for Employing Baby-sitters

New parents are usually novice employers of baby-sitters
as well. Make the experience go well all around by doing
the following:

- Meet the person before you engage her services, and
  get recommendations from several reliable sources.
  Feeling comfortable with your sitter is the keystone to
  everything going well.

- Establish ground rules up front: No visitors; help yourself to whatever food you like, whatever.
- Leave contact information regarding where you are going and when, as well as the name of your pediatrician and the doctor's after-hours emergency number.
- Don't require the sitter to do much other than look after your child. That should be her sole priority. If you need cleaning or cooking done, hire a maid or a caterer. (Exception: If the sitter is a full-time child-care worker, you may negotiate for her to perform a reasonable amount of housework, to be performed while the baby naps.)
- Let the sitter know what time you will return. Don't be late.
- Discuss in advance how the sitter will get home and whether transportation (a lift, a cab) is necessary.

How often is it cool to call a baby-sitter to check up on the baby?

Because you are the parents, you set the tone. If you want to call every hour on the hour, that's your prerogative. The baby-sitter should not feel that this is intrusive or a sign of being considered untrustworthy.

Before you dial as frequently as every hour, however, realize that you are away from home either to work or to have fun. You won't be able to accomplish much of either if you dwell excessively on the safety and happiness of your infant. Anyway, your child is probably quite safe and quite happy, since you have left him or her in the guardianship of a baby-sitter whom you trust.

If you do not trust the sitter, get yourself home right away and find one you do. If you do trust the sitter, check in once just to satisfy your own peace of mind, and then force yourself to get on with your day.

Do free-market rules apply to baby-sitters—that is, can I lure a friend's sitter away by promising better pay?
This is, of course, America, land of supply and demand, equal opportunity, and all that. It's certainly legal to lure away a friend's highly recommended baby-sitter, though not recommended if one wishes to retain the friend.

If the sitter does not have a standing agreement with your friend, on the other hand, you are free to call that sitter for her services. You don't need to clear the date first with your friend. The sitter can work for both of you as she sees fit.

ADVICE

How do I respond to the unwanted advice of perfect strangers about baby care?
Some strangers can't help themselves. Babies are magnets for check-pinchers and toe-ticklers and advice-dolers. And the first two are actually more annoying, since they involve physical contact between a perfect stranger and your precious baby.

Rehearse a patient smile. When someone nags about how you've dressed your child or what you're feeding him or whether or not she's wearing a hat—and inevitably, if you take your child out in public, someone will—flash the smile and move on. Or say, "Thanks for your concern, but she's just fine."

When one woman I know was confronted by such unsolicited advice, she cheerfully asked each lecturer for his or her name and phone number. "Why do you want that?"

they'd ask. "Well, my lawyer advised me to write down all the people who told me how to raise my baby so that I could more easily go back and sue them if their advice didn't work so well."

Quick Comebacks to the Curious

If you thought pregnancy made you a target for rude and nosy comments, wait 'til the baby arrives. There's no end to what some people will come out with.

When They Say . . .	*You Can Say . . .*
"She certainly doesn't look like you."	"No, I'm much taller."
"Isn't she cute." (But she's a boy.)	"His name is Michael."
"Isn't he adorable." (But he's a girl.)	"Her name is Michele."
"Where's her hat?"	"It's in her bag, thanks."
"I think he's too hot."	"He's not complaining."
"Are you the grand-mother?"	"No, I'm the mother." (Don't feel embarrassed—wait for the other party to grovel their apologies.)

When They Say...	*You Can Say...*
"When are you having the next one?"	"Not today, I'm afraid."

GETTING AWAY

When should we first go away overnight without our baby?
That's entirely a personal matter. Some parents feel comfortable leaving on extended trips, in qualified care, when their baby is still just weeks old. (British royalty does it all the time.) Others wait years before they spend a night away. Let your conscience, and the availability of trustworthy care, be your guide.

How should we respond to criticism that we don't get out enough now that we're parents?
Listen carefully before you dismiss the comment outright. If it's your childless old pals who are doing the complaining, they may not be able to relate to your change of heart. Many new parents are surprised to discover that they suddenly, somehow, no longer miss seeing first-run movies or eating out at their favorite restaurants. At least at first, babies really are that absorbing. If it's your parents or a close friend who is volunteering to help watch the baby, they may have your concerns more at stake than their own. Perhaps they see signs of depression or marital discord—which are both common side effects of new parenthood. In that event, perhaps taking a break would do you good.

All you need to say immediately is, "Thanks for your concern." Whether or not you act is up to you.

ONE UP-MOM-SHIP

What's the best way to react to competitive parents who compare my child's progress to their own?
Because first-time parents haven't been down that road of life before, it's natural to want to do a certain amount of signpost checking: Is my baby growing properly? Hitting the major milestones on time? Sure lots of this information can be found in books, but there's nothing like comparing notes with other mothers, particularly those whose children are the same age, or slightly older. This sort of exchange is perfectly normal, when carried out in the innocent spirit of information-gathering and marveling.

It can quickly devolve into a nastier type of one-upmanship, however. Danger signs:

- The mother who continuously offers up "I can top that" stories
- The mother who reports signs of an advanced IQ in a baby who can't even sit up yet
- The mother who puts down another's baby, even in veiled terms ("She's awfully clingy, isn't she?")
- Conversations that always include the words "Well *my* baby can . . ."

Avoid these women. It will only get worse.

MOTHERS' GROUPS

Can I invite myself into a group of mothers that I know congregate in my neighborhood?

Inviting oneself to a mom's group at someone's home borders on the presumptuous, like inviting yourself to a book club or other private regular gathering. (If it's a public gathering run by a local organization, that's a different story. You don't need an invitation to drop by.) The thoughtful thing for the neighborhood moms to do would be to notice you waddling around the neighborhood before the baby is born and to mention their get-togethers then.

But even if this hasn't happened, don't despair. Moms need other moms, so you don't have to stand on ceremony. Take the lead yourself by inviting one or two of the mothers to your house with their babies. Chances are good that your hospitality will be reciprocated and you'll become one of the gang.

What do I do if I feel excluded by the local mother's group because I'm older than everyone else?

It's unlikely that the other mothers are intentionally shunning you because of your age. But it may be that you lack the same social references (music, socioeconomic status) that can make for an easier rapport. It's possible that an older mom might intimidate younger mothers, who mistakenly infer that she must know more about motherhood because she is more mature or has more work experience.

It also may be possible for an older mom to imagine slights that just aren't there because she is self-conscious about her age. Most new moms, when thrown together, find plenty to talk about just focusing on such mundane new realities as feeding schedules and when babies roll over.

You might just be more comfortable with a different group of women. Look for parents with similar life experiences, such as other moms who work. Through your doctor's office or a local parenting network it may be possible to find a mother's group especially for older first-time parents.

You can gain insight and support (if not a ready-made baby-sitting co-op) by joining an on-line mother's group. There are dozens of them on the Internet.

On-Line Moms' Group Tips

To get the most out of your mother's group:

- Find the right fit. Troll through several sites to find the best match for you. For example, you might prefer a site that advocates or focuses on attachment-style parenting, Christian parenthood, health issues only, lesbian motherhood, or parenting multiples. There's definitely something for everyone.
- Consider regional groups. You might want to connect with e-pals who live near you, in order to later meet for off-line mother's groups or baby-sitting co-ops.
- Don't use all caps in your postings. Online, it's akin to shouting.
- Catch the drift first. Read back several messages so that you don't introduce a question that everyone else already finished dissecting two weeks ago.
- Learn the lingo. "DH" is mom-group slang for "dear husband," "SAHM" means "stay-at-home mom," and so on.
- Be supportive, rather than critical. Just because you can't see your fellow moms face-to-face is no excuse to slam their opinions and practices. Most moms go on-line to find kindred spirits or solutions to problems.

CHILDBIRTH-CLASS REUNIONS

Is it customary to have a reunion of the couples in your childbirth class, and who organizes this event if so?

A childbirth-education class reunion is common in some areas, and among some instructors, and alien to others. Couples who attend numerous childbirth-education classes together sometimes forge strong bonds. It can be interesting to see what all those other people who nervously practiced breathing and massage with you now look like as parents. A benefit to such an event is that new mothers get to network with other new mothers.

Some instructors routinely plan such an event for their students, although because they teach many classes in a year, such women are a rarity. More typically, they may plant the idea for a reunion with their students, and ask everyone to share their names and addresses (and due dates) with one another, if they like, should one couple want to take the lead later.

A reunion is usually scheduled six or eight weeks after everyone can be expected to have delivered. Depending on the class size, you can invite the others by telephone or send a simple card. It's equally okay to invite couples or just the mothers. (Babies, of course, are required to be on hand!) No one expects grand entertainment from new parents. Keep the event simple, such as a tea or a potluck lunch.

If one or two connections persist as the result of such a gathering, it's a bonus. But the hosts should not be disappointed if the group does not stay in touch, nor is any guest obligated to reciprocate, since this is in essence, a group of strangers who have been brought together through unusual circumstances.

Where the Moms Are

Looking for ways to meet other new mothers? Consider the following:

- Join a health club. Many YMCAs and spas have nurseries for young children.
- Look for support groups near you. Surf the web or ads in local parenting publications for national networks that might have branches near you, such as MOMS Club (Moms Offering Moms Support), Mothers at Home, FEMALE (Formerly Employed Mothers at the Leading Edge), La Leche League International, and the National Association of Mothers' Centers.
- Investigate parents' groups at your local place of worship or your pediatrician's office.
- Start your own support group. Post a message for other mothers in your neighborhood community center or library.

FIRST BIRTHDAY

What's the protocol for the first birthday party?
Realize this key thing: The first birthday is for you, more than your child. Your baby (okay, fledgling toddler) doesn't know a birthday cake from a mud pie. He may enjoy the fuss, but he's certainly not expecting any. Nor will he remember it.

That's not to say you shouldn't celebrate. By all means, do! You've both reached a big milestone together! Most parents have at least a cake and ice cream, and sing a round of "Happy

Birthday." Be more ambitious than that at your own risk. Not only are jugglers, ponies, and magicians expensive, they may not be appreciated by your newly minted one-year-old. Little ones have been known to cry in fear at the festivities—or just fall asleep.

The bottom line: Do what feels right for you. Just don't expect too much.

What should I do if my child has a December birthday?

The first year or two, before true birthday awareness sets in, your child won't care. Have a small celebration for the birthday and then celebrate the holiday in your usual fashion.

As your child grows older, you may want to stretch the distance between these two big events in order to avoid celebration overload and to make your child feel like his or her special day is truly special. Some families celebrate the child's "half-birthday" with a summer party. Others inch the birthday festivities up to October or November, or push them back to January or February.

It's also perfectly appropriate to play the birthdays as they lie. One family decorates their Christmas tree with balloons, streamers, candles, and other birthday artifacts until their child's big day in mid-month; then they switch to Yuletide ornaments. Another clan looks for birthday-party venues that are low on Christmas decorations, such as indoor playlands or roller rinks.

And be sure to let your child know that he or she is the best present *you* ever received.

Birthday Memory Making

Your baby's first birthday is a major milestone for both of you. A few suggestions to capture the event for posterity:

- Schedule a portrait. A good way to remember to get periodic formal photographs of your child is to plan to have them taken on (or during the week of) his or her birthday.
- Send "you are there" thank-you cards. Take several photographs of the classic first-birthday-cake scene. Use them to decorate notecards to thank family and friends who sent presents but couldn't be there in person. (Many catalogs sell folded photo cards with spaces for placing a three-by-five-inch or four-by-six-inch snapshot.)
- Start a height record. Now that she can stand up pretty well, mark your child's height on a designated wall (or special board or paper you can buy for this purpose) and update the measurement every six months.
- Snap your child wearing a special adult-sized piece of clothing: a sweatshirt from your alma mater, a bathing suit, Daddy's old football jersey, a fancy dress. Do the same thing every year and watch your baby grow into it.
- Or shoot an annual photo of your child standing in front of a tree that you plant in honor of her first birthday. Watch them grow together.
- Make a point to update the baby book with a quick summary of the birthday party, recent accomplishments, and other details you always mean to record but never get around to.

- Borrow a Native American tradition and start a blessings bag. In a cloth pouch, place sentimental objects relating to family members—Grandma's thimble, Daddy's tie, and so on. Include a written explanation of each item. Add to it as your child grows.

- Start a birthday video. Tape the crucial minutes of the party (blowing out the candle, digging into the cake) at the beginning of a new videotape. Mark the tape "Birthday Video" and store it away. Every year, bring it out on your child's birthday to add a few more minutes of festivities.

- Write a letter to your child. Review the year—her milestones, changes, big events, and so on. Let her know how much she means to you. Seal the envelope and put it away in a special box or large envelope. Do the same every year on her birthday. When she's eighteen, you'll have an extraspecial gift to give her.

14

Great Gifts

What's the perfect present for the occasion? Here are some time-tested ideas for various birth-related circumstances.

Remember that gifts for special occasions deserve special wrappings, too. They don't have to be expensive. Even the simplest ready-made gift bags, trussed with colored tissue paper and ribbons, add a special touch to a gift for mother or baby. For extra festiveness, tie a cute rattle or stuffed toy onto the ribbon of the package. Another idea: Save the newspapers from the day the baby is born, and use them as gift wrap.

A nice idea for thank-yous: Photograph the baby wearing or using the item. The giver will appreciate the gesture, and if you order double prints, you keep the other, providing a great excuse to keep on snapping pictures of your fast-changing babe.

EXPECTANT MOTHER PICK-ME-UPS

Maybe you're visiting a friend in the last weeks of her pregnancy. Of you want to send something from afar. These gifts celebrate her new stage of life and help make the weeks zip along:

- Favorite herbal tea and pretty cup or mug
- Pampering gift certificate (for manicure, haircut, etc.)

- Books about baby care, baby names
- Humor book about pregnancy or parenthood
- Journal to record thoughts about pregnancy
- A "cravings basket" filled with her favorite snacks
- Jar of pickles and a certificate for a local ice-cream parlor
- A body pillow
- Maternity clothes loaners (she may be grateful for something fresh to wear as the seasons change)
- Nursing nightgown (with special concealed openings; can be worn now and is also useful later)
- Nursing blouse (see above)
- Humorous T-shirt (size XL or maternity) with a slogan such as "This woman deserves a party" or "Look but don't touch."
- Pretty scarf
- Fun socks
- Slippers with nonskid soles
- Beautiful bathrobe (to wear now and later)
- Armload of the latest magazines
- Movie cassettes and popcorn
- Relaxing music
- Massage lotion for sore feet
- Bath salts
- Small, pretty pillow to support her back
- Flowers or a plant in a pretty vase or basket
- Stationery (for all the thank-you notes she'll be needing to write)
- Gift-of-the-month club (fruit, flowers, pizzas, socks—if given for a full year, it will last past the baby's arrival)
- Weekend away (for couples, a mid-pregnancy escape may be the last chance you have for a while)
- IOUs for running errands, doing laundry, and so on
- A copy of this book

BABY SHOWER

Shower presents are traditionally inexpensive baby-care items to help feather the growing family's nest. The giving of larger items (strollers, baby swings), by individuals or by a group that has pooled resources, is a recent development. Some useful ideas:

- Baby clothes (especially in sizes larger than three months): onesies, undershirts, booties, hat-and-sweater set, sleepers, sleep-sacques with gathered bottoms, playclothes—especially for girls, who tend to be showered with dressy items. Drawstring gowns (also called sacs) are wonderful for newborns because they simplify diaper changing. *Presentation ideas*: If you buy several items, present them attached to a clothesline that can be held out or strung up at the shower. Or get together with a friend and pack the clothes in a new hamper.
- Soft baby shoes and socks
- Beautiful baby bonnet or other infant hats
- Bunting (for cool weather)
- Bibs (small juice size and larger ones; everyday and fancy)
- Baby bottles, bottle warmer, dishwasher container for nipples and rings
- Melamine baby dishes and sippy cups
- Picture frame
- Simple baby toys (rattles, stuffed or musical toy, baby-safe mirror, blocks)
- Baby's first teddy bear
- "Knotty doll" made of soft fabric
- Infant "gym" (special toy bar, some with a mat)

- Activity mat
- Newborn-sized diapers
- Receiving blankets
- Stroller blanket (slightly heavier than receiving blanket; Polarfleece is both soft and warm)
- Nice fitted crib sheets (flannel, 100% cotton, or stretchy cotton)
- Bassinet or cradle sheets
- Cloth diapers (can be used as burp cloths or lap pads)
- Baby toiletry items (nail clippers, scissors, thermometer, nice baby shampoos or soaps, brush-and-comb set) in a diaper pail, diaper bag, or other useful container
- Basket of child-safe items (outlet plugs, drawer locks, doorknob covers, toilet lock, gate)
- Commuter's box: Clear box filled with travel-with-baby necessities, such as a rearview mirror to see the backseat, a terry-cloth head support, a shade for the car window, a car-seat protector, plastic toy links for attaching a rattle or toy to the car seat, travel-size baby wipes, and so on.
- Infant-clothes hangers
- Baby bathtub or tub seat and bath toys
- Sponge pad (for sitting on in tub)
- Hooded towels and infant washcloths
- Diaper bag (beware that this is a very personal item; give thought to the mother-to-be's tastes)
- Diaper disposal method (diaper pail or type that automatically wraps individual diapers in plastic)
- Newborn or size-one diapers
- Large supply of baby wipes
- Changing-table cover pad
- Car-seat cover or head support
- Humidifier
- Crib light
- Food grinder (for baby food)

- Baby book
- Baby photo album
- Classic children's books like *Goodnight Moon*, *Hush Little Baby*, *Time for Bed*, *Harold and the Purple Crayon*, nursery rhymes.
- Other baby board books (look for popular children's characters such as Winnie the Pooh, Barney, Teletubbies, Clifford the Big Red Dog)
- Subscription to a parenting magazine
- Cassette tapes or CDs of Lullabies
- Piggy bank
- Growth chart, baby book, developmental calendar (for recording baby milestones)
- Baby photo album and lots of film
- Nursery décor (framed print, appliqué pillow, nightlight)
- Nursing shawl
- Soft infant carrier for babywearing (sling style)
- Bouncy seat
- Monitor
- Mobile
- Music box

GIFTS FOR DAD-TO-BE

At coed showers, it can be fun to single out the expectant father with gifts like these:

- "I Love Daddy" bib
- Relaxing music (to listen to during labor and after)
- Books about fatherhood (check the parenting section at any bookstore)
- Cigars

- Blank videocassette tapes or film (especially if he's a camera buff)
- T-shirt with the words "Old Block" and baby T-shirt or onesie that says "Chip"
- Humorous new-parent "Survival Kit": earplugs, snack foods (for labor), aspirin, instant coffee, No-Doz, rubber gloves (for diapers)

Birth Bouquets

Send flowers with special meaning to new parents. The traditional birthflowers are as follows:

- January: carnation
- February: violet
- March: daffodil
- April: sweet pea
- May: Lily of the valley
- June: rose
- July: delphinium
- August: gladiolus
- September: aster
- October: marigold
- November: chrysanthemum
- December: pointsettia

BIRTH OR ADOPTION

Nowadays, the line between a shower gift and one given to celebrate and commemorate a child's arrival has become blurred. Traditionally, gifts given at birth or adoption are more lavish or lasting than shower presents. Or you can use your imagination to come up with something appropriately special.

While showers are not usually held for second-or later-borns, it's correct to bestow a gift upon the birth of such children.

Sample birth or adoption gifts:

- Silver cup engraved with baby's name and birthdate
- Silver baby spoon engraved with baby's initial
- Silver porringer
- Silver picture frame engraved with baby's name
- Silver rattle or teething ring
- Silver comb-and-brush set
- Commemorative ceramic baby cup
- Carved or painted keepsake box for baby's mementos, decorated with baby's name
- A piece of jewelry with the child's birthstone
- Piece of heirloom jewelry (grandmother's locket, grandfather's watch)
- Keepsake crib quilt
- Personalized baby blanket
- Cross-stitch, embroidery, or other handmade item bearing baby's name and birthdate (pillow, wall hanging, framed piece)
- A letter to the child, to be read on his or her sixteenth birthday; high-school graduation, or other special day (ideal from a grandparent or parent)

- Hand-knit items (baby sweater, blanket)
- Hand-smocked baby gown
- Nice quality photo album
- A filled-out memory book from Grandma and/or Grandpa. (Look for these fill-in-the-blank books in bookstores or children's shops; include Xeroxes of old family photos and documents.)
- A time capsule (including newspapers, magazines, and other memorabilia from the birth date, sealed and to be opened on the child's eighteenth birthday)
- Hand-sewn cloth baby book (such as of ABCs, animals, different textures and shapes)
- First piggy bank
- Moses basket (for carrying a newborn) with fabric liner and matching quilt
- Savings bond
- Money earmarked for college tuition
- Set of newly minted coins of the year of the baby's birth
- Gift certificate to baby store, photography studio, catalog
- "IOU" coupons for helper services (from a close friend or relative—for baby-sitting, grocery shopping, laundry services, rides to the pediatrician, tea and sympathy, and so on)
- Warehouse-size boxes of paper plates, cups, and disposable silverware to make the new parents' first days dishwashing-free
- Decorative small rug, for nursery
- A hope chest (stock it with items for baby's future: a first-birthday outfit, fine wine for baby's wedding, a family heirloom)
- Set of silver or pewter decorative birthday-candle holders (featuring children's theme such as circus figurines or Beatrix Potter animals)

- Decorative family tree, perhaps suitable for framing
- Hand-painted child's chair or rocker
- Step-stool (hand-painted or with name carved into it)
- Wooden rocking horse
- Well-made wooden toy train
- Large piece of baby equipment: Car seat, stroller, high chair, exer-saucer, playpen, Portacrib, swing, rocking chair with footstool. (Note: Do not give infant walkers, unless they are the new type that are not mobile. Infant walkers are a leading cause of accidents.)

Birthstones

Gifts relating to the traditional calendar of birthstones can add a special dimension to a gift. The father might give the mother a piece of jewelry representing the month of the baby's birth. Or the baby may be given a small necklace, to be worn when she is older. Wearing one's birthstone is said to bring luck. Traditional birthstones (and their corresponding colors and meanings) are:

- January: Garnet (deep red; constancy)
- February: Amethyst (purple; sincerity)
- March: Aquamarine (pale blue; truth)
- April: Diamond (white; innocence)
- May: Emerald (green; happiness)
- June: Pearl (white; health)
- July: Ruby (red; love)
- August: Peridot (light green; felicity)

- September: Sapphire (deep blue; wisdom)
- October: Opal (iridescent; hope)
- November: Topaz (yellow; fidelity)
- December: Turquoise (bright sky blue; success)

CHRISTENING

The godparents and close family members normally give a special gift at baptism. Others invited to a christening, who may have already given baby gifts, may give a small token although this is not necessary. In some cultures, this is one occasion when it's not only acceptable, but traditional, to give cash (or a savings bond) to fund a bank account for the child. Classic baby gifts of lasting value are also appropriate, as are the following religious-themed gifts:

- A Bible (children's or adult version; with date of christening inscribed inside; some brides later carry their baptismal Bible down the aisle)
- Cross necklace
- Crucifix for wall display
- Rosary beads (for Catholic)
- Religious-themed children's books
- Religious-themed children's videos (such as Veggie Tales)
- Beautiful white blanket to be used at christening.

BRIS

The *bris* is a convenient time to bestow a welcome-baby gift. Especially suitable is a present that has special significance regarding the baby's Jewish heritage, though you're not limited to religious gifts. Some choices in addition to the usual baby gifts:

- Money
- Handmade infant skullcap (to be worn during *bris*)
- *Kiddish* cup
- Heirloom-quality dreidel (silver, ceramic, carved wood)
- Jewish children's books
- Jewish children's audio-or videotapes
- Wood blocks spelling the child's Hebrew name
- Baby's Hebrew name embroidered on a baby blanket
- Portrait, scrapbook, or other mementos about the person for whom the child is named
- Jewish artwork for the nursery

GIFTS FOR OLDER SIBLINGS

It's thoughtful (though not necessary) to bring along a gift for an older child when you go to visit a new baby. Children ages two-and-a-half to seven or eight benefit most from such a gesture. Younger than that, and they may not understand much of what's going on, and children older than eight are usually secure enough not to feel displaced by all the excitement of a new baby. Certainly, though, a token will be welcomed by a sibling of any age. Such gifts need not be expensive. If they underscore siblinghood or a growing independence, so much the better. Examples (both large and small) include:

- T-shirts or buttons that say, "I'm the Big Brother/Sister."
- Books about babies
- Baby doll

- Baby doll accoutrements: soft carrier, bottles, diapers, umbrella stroller
- Disposable camera
- Brag book
- Cassette player or tapes
- Small toy
- Stuffed animal "baby," such as a lamb, a kitten, a puppy
- Puzzle
- Box of animal crackers
- Special candy, such as an old-fashioned giant lollipop
- Stickers and sticker book
- Art kit (markers, safety scissors, paper tape)
- Mylar balloons (these present less of a choking hazard than traditional balloons because they don't burst into pieces).
- Tricycle (or other toy that underscores a preschooler's advanced skills, relative to the baby)
- Wagon

FIRST BIRTHDAY

A baby's first birthday is a huge milestone for the parents—though the honoree is apt to be unawares. Gifts given to mark this occasion are therefore mostly for the parent's benefit, and one can get away with giving a one-year-old more useful items than he's liable to welcome just a year later at his second birthday. Consider things like:

- A contribution to baby's college fund (with a full seventeen years to go, the interest will compound impressively)
  ⌐lothing in larger sizes
    ⌐y album made of highlights of the past year

- Blank photo album (for recording the coming years)
- Blank videocassette tapes
- Shoes (welcome for emerging walkers)
- Board books (most parents should begin reading regularly to their child now, if they haven't already)
- Videos for the very young (Teletubbies, Spot, Barney)
- Push toys (to encourage walking)
- Sippy cups, melamine place settings of children's dishes, child-scaled spoons and forks
- First ride-on toys
- Stacking cups or rings
- Toy telephone or bank
- Blocks (large-sized wood, or cloth or cardboard; or plastic Duplo-style)

About the Author

PAULA SPENCER, the mother of four, is a contributing editor of *Parenting* and *Woman's Day* magazines and has written extensively about parenthood.

Send your pregnancy- and birth-related customs or your questions about maternity manners to her at Plaspencer@aol.com or care of P.O. Box 5558, Knoxville, TN 37928.